ATOPIC SKIN DISEASE

A MANUAL FOR PRACTITIONERS

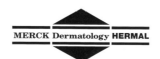

ATOPIC SKIN DISEASE

A MANUAL FOR PRACTITIONERS

Christopher Bridgett

Consultant Psychiatrist, Chelsea & Westminster Hospital, London, UK

Peter Norén

Consultant Dermatologist, Uppsala, Sweden

and

Richard Staughton

Consultant Dermatologist, Chelsea & Westminster Hospital, London, UK

WRIGHTSON BIOMEDICAL PUBLISHING LTD

Petersfield, UK and Bristol, PA, USA

ATOPIC SKIN DISEASE:
A Manual for Practitioners
First published in Great Britain by
Wrightson Biomedical Publishing Ltd

Editorial Office:
Wrightson Biomedical Publishing Ltd
Ash Barn House, Winchester Road,
Stroud, Petersfield, Hampshire
GU32 3PN
Telephone: 44 +1730 265647
Fax: 44 +1730 260368

A CIP catalogue record for this title is
available from the British Library

A CIP catalog record for this title is
available from the Library of Congress

ISBN 1 871816 32 7

Photomicrographs by Dr N.D. Fancis,
Charing Cross and Westminster
Medical School, London, UK
Cartoons by Mats Böllner,
Helsingborg, Sweden
Text design by Russell Townsend,
Bognor Regis, UK
Composition by Scribe Design,
Gillingham, Kent, UK
Printed and Bound by
Butler & Tanner, Frome, UK

CONTENTS

PREFACE

In the summer of 1989 at the International Congress on Dermatology and Psychiatry in Leeds, UK, Richard Staughton introduced Peter Norén to Christopher Bridgett. This led to a fruitful discussion of the work done by Peter Norén and his colleagues at the University Hospital in Uppsala, Sweden, where they had introduced habit reversal to the management of atopic skin disease in 1984. Our subsequent collaboration led to the introduction of 'The Combined Approach' for atopic eczema at the Daniel Turner Clinic, Westminster Hospital, London, in the autumn of 1989. As we gained experience and gathered further clinical data, we were able to report on our work at the Congress on Dermatology and Psychiatry in Florence in 1991 and in Amsterdam in 1995.

Success with patients has led to pressure to promulgate the technique. The handbook for patients has been developed into a training video for professionals. Now this manual allows the method to be mastered with ease by appropriately trained health service practitioners, both doctors and nurses, working in primary and secondary health care settings. The Combined Approach is highly effective, and can radically improve the quality of life of the majority of patients with long-term atopic skin disease.

In our work we have learnt a great deal by listening to our patients. We wish to acknowledge their contribution to this volume, and to express our gratitude to Christina Funnel and her colleagues at the National Eczema Society, London, for all the help and encouragement they have given us.

CHRISTOPHER BRIDGETT, PETER NORÉN
AND RICHARD STAUGHTON,
JULY 1996

FOREWORD

The practice of medicine, and of dermatology in particular revolves around the consultation and good communication. This book is a testament to effective communication, not only between two dermatologists, one practising in Sweden and the other in London, but also between them and an interested and motivated psychiatrist.

The establishment of the European Society for Dermatology and Psychiatry ultimately brought the three authors together and I am sure innumerable patients with atopic eczema will benefit from The Combined Approach advocated in this novel and important new book.

I hope this work will be read by as wide an audience as possible, and not only by doctors, dermatologists and nurses, but also by patients. There is no doubt that The Combined Approach to eczema described here is effective and so will improve the quality of life for many patients with atopic eczema.

I think this book has every chance of becoming a classic in the dermatological literature and I am sure many patients will be grateful to the authors for all the time and effort they have put into producing it.

J. A. COTTERILL MD BSc FRCP
Medical Director, Lasercare Clinics,
and Consultant Dermatologist

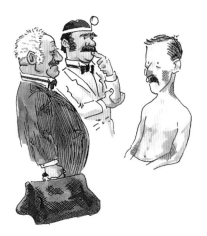

1

INTRODUCTION

1.1 Atopic Skin Disease and The Combined Approach

Eczema and dermatitis

Eczema and dermatitis are terms that are now used synonymously for a particular type of skin inflammation. Histologically eczema is characterised by the epidermis being swollen with fluid: **spongiosis**.

Atopic skin disease and Besnier's prurigo

Atopy is a constitutional state associated with a vulnerability to develop asthma, hay fever and eczema. **Atopic skin disease** is a term also used synonymously with **atopic eczema** and **atopic dermatitis** (Fig 1.1); it can embrace not only the various stages of atopic eczema, but also its various complications.

While atopic eczema shows recognisable clinical patterns at different ages, a most striking behavioural characteristic throughout is **scratching**. Scratching of the skin begins as a reflex response to the **itch** of eczema. In one of the earliest accounts differentiating atopic eczema from other skin conditions, the French physician Besnier called it simply 'the itch' (prurigo). For many years atopic eczema was therefore known as **Besnier's prurigo** (Plate 1.1).

The Combined Approach

The need for a fresh approach to the management of atopic eczema prompted a collaboration in the 1980s between colleagues at the University Hospital in Uppsala, Sweden (Melin *et al.*, 1986). Their work has been subsequently developed at the Chelsea and Westminster

---

Fig 1.1 Synonymous Terms

Atopic skin disease
•
Atopic dermatitis
•
Atopic eczema
•
Besnier's prurigo

Plate 1.1 Ernest Besnier 1831–1909 gave an early account of atopic skin disease: Besnier's prurigo.

1

Fig 1.2 Key Message

*The Combined
Approach*

Optimal conventional

treatment

plus

Behaviour modification

Fig 1.3 The Atopic Triad

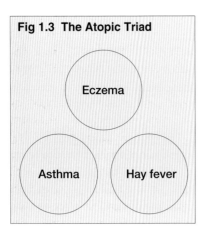

Hospital in London, where the term 'The Combined Approach' was coined to emphasise the bringing together of conventional dermatological treatments with a set of psychological treatments that both optimise the effectiveness of the topical remedies and seek to eliminate the self-damaging behaviours that otherwise complicate atopic dermatitis (Fig 1.2).

1.2 Atopy and Atopic Skin Disease

Atopy

The term atopy is a descriptive word meaning 'strange disease' that was introduced in the early 1920s to encompass that group of patients prone to asthma, eczema, infantile food hypersensitivity and hay fever (seasonal rhinitis) (Fig 1.3). The allergic tendency was seen to run in families, with affected individuals experiencing one or any combination or succession of these clinical conditions. While eczema is the main skin manifestation of atopy, transient urticarial swellings can develop around the mouth associated with infantile food allergies, and severe insect bite reactions are said to be more common in atopic individuals.

The nature of atopy

Despite atopic conditions being common, much remains to be discovered about both the mode of inheritance, and the allergic mechanism involved. Although severe cases of atopic eczema have obvious unifying clinical features, there is no one diagnostic physical sign or laboratory test to aid recognition of the milder condition. Thus although some authorities define atopy as the ability to develop particular antibodies in response to certain environmental allergens, a small but significant percentage of individuals with 'typical' atopic eczema do not show this immune reaction, using the laboratory tests currently available. Atopy therefore remains essentially a clinical concept.

The origin of atopy

As atopy is common, it may have a useful function. There is evidence that atopy is associated with a resistance to parasitic infestation. It is only in the recent past

Plate 1.2 House dust mites 'grazing'. The large slab in front of them is a shed skin cell (house dust), their staple diet.

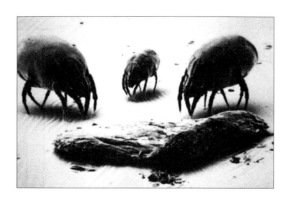

that Western man has lost the parasitic load his predecessors carried. In Papua New Guinea the intestinal parasites found in atopics with asthma are significantly reduced compared with those found in non-atopics.

A low parasitic load means better nutrition and more chance of survival to maturity and breeding. Thus the gene associated with this advantage is conserved, and becomes more common.

In the western world, the allergens that are engaged by this defence mechanism are characteristic of modern living, namely allergens trapped in the modern dwelling – the faecal pellets of the house dust mite and the mite itself (*Dermatophagoides pteronyssimus*) (Plate 1.2), which feeds on shed human skin, and epidermal cells (**dander**) shed from domesticated animals, e.g. cats and dogs. We have perhaps exchanged protection from parasites for allergic disease (Fig 1.4).

Fig 1.4 Atopy

> A common state

> No single biological marker

> A **disadvantage** for the advantaged?

Prevalence

In most western countries clinical experience has suggested for some time that the prevalence of asthma, hay fever and eczema are all increasing. Published studies confirm this impression, though such work is hampered by the lack of hard diagnostic criteria for these conditions.

Fig 1.5 Prevalence

- 25–30% population genetically atopic

- 5–15% school children ⎫
- 2–10% adults ⎬ atopic eczema

While 25–30% of a population may be genetically atopic, the prevalence of particular conditions is dictated by the intensity of exposure to environmental allergens. Atopic eczema is a common disease affecting 5–15% of school children and 2–10% of adults (Fig 1.5). Patients with atopic skin disease account for some 15% of all referrals to dermatologists and about 30% of dermatological consultations in general practice. About 50% of infants with atopic eczema later develop asthma, and hay fever.

Genetics

Although there is a clear tendency for atopy to run in families, the precise mode of inheritance is unknown. Non-atopic parents do not usually have atopic children. In large families it is possible to see that atopy is transmitted vertically from one generation to the next. In one careful survey in the 1990s, it was found that of marriages in which one partner was atopic about half the children were affected, and about three quarters when both parents were. These figures are consistent with an autosomal dominant inheritance, but as 10% of affected children did not have an atopic parent, penetrance is not complete. Current research suggests a relevant gene on chromosome 11.

Natural history of atopic skin disease

Atopic eczema most often starts between the third and sixth month of life. In only a quarter of cases does the disease persist into childhood, and generally a spontaneous remission occurs before or during adolescence. Only a small proportion continue into adulthood (Fig 1.6). The history then is one of long-standing disease which remits and relapses according to a wide variety of social, physical and psychological factors (pp. 105–106). The condition then tends to disappear in middle age.

A minority of infants with atopic eczema that shows complete remission in childhood later re-present in their late teens or twenties with severe disease. This may be associated with important changes in circumstances, such as leaving home and starting independent life, either in further education or employment.

Such severely affected adults can be in most need of The Combined Approach. Their quality of life is often adversely affected, with self image, confidence and in particular sexual life all being profoundly compromised.

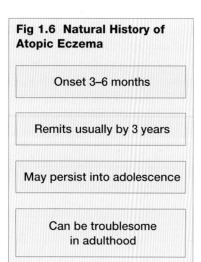

Fig 1.6 Natural History of Atopic Eczema

Onset 3–6 months

Remits usually by 3 years

May persist into adolescence

Can be troublesome in adulthood

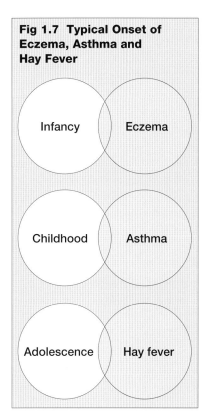

Fig 1.7 Typical Onset of Eczema, Asthma and Hay Fever

Infancy — Eczema

Childhood — Asthma

Adolescence — Hay fever

The relationship between eczema, food intolerance, asthma and hay fever

At any one time one condition tends to prevail, and this seems to be age-related (Fig 1.7). Eczema and food intolerances usually come first, between three and six months of age. Food intolerance wanes rapidly. A very few patients retain real and sometimes potentially life threatening reactions to certain foods, e.g. nuts and fish. It is important to note that eczema rarely accompanies such hypersensitivity.

Eczema remits naturally before the age of three in 75% of children. Asthma starts a little later than eczema, peaking at about four years. Eczema and asthma commonly co-exist. Active treatment of asthma with inhaled steroids and bronchodilators has little influence on eczema severity. A course of systemic steroids for a severe asthmatic attack may however improve eczema temporarily, and a course of antibiotic given for the chest may also benefit the skin, both by reducing the staphylococcal population, and through the anti-inflammatory properties of the antibiotic.

Hay fever is often the last of the atopic triad to emerge, usually in the early teens. Although it is commonly caused by grass pollen, it can be triggered by house dust mites, and animal dander. Occasionally these allergens trigger eczema, asthma and hay fever simultaneously — an atopic 'full-house'.

Diagnosis

The presentation of atopic skin disease varies with age (Fig 1.8), but the results of scratching and rubbing the skin are the invariable unifying characteristics. Plates 1.3 to 1.14 illustrate the diagnostically significant physical features of atopic skin disease in babies, children and adults. Babies irritably roll about, rubbing their skin against the mattress and the sides of the cot (Plate 1.3). Red, swollen and broken skin is seen over the **convexities** of the body, sparing protected areas such as eye-sockets, the gutters around the nostrils, and the skin covered by the nappy. Worst affected areas are the cheeks, forehead, occiput (where the hair is usually rubbed away) and the external convexities of the upper arms.

Motor development brings with it the facility for **directional scratching**. The dermatitis is now predom-

Fig 1.8 Common Sites of Chronic Infantile Eczema

Youngest	Older
Cheeks	Eyelids
Forehead	Earlobes
Occiput	Wrists
Upper arms	Ankles

5

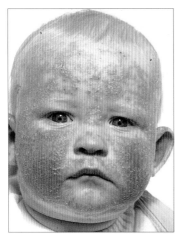

Plate 1.3   Atopic baby's face. A restless, irritable baby rolls about in its cot rubbing the convexities of forehead and cheeks against the cot floor and sides. Note the sparing within the eye sockets and gutters alongside the nose.

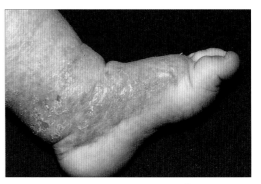

Plate 1.4   Atopic baby's foot. Severe swelling, thickening and reddening of the skin caused by friction of the foot again opposing leg. Note sparing in sites protected by the shoe.

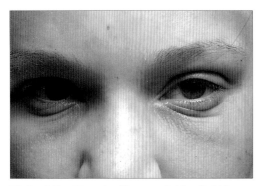

Plate 1.5   Dennie–Morgan folds. Rubbing around the eyes causes thickening of the skin with accentuation of the natural skin creases. This gives the appearance of an extra fold below the eye.

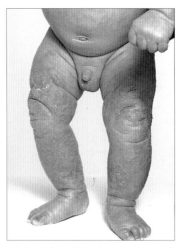

Plate 1.6   Atopic eczema affecting the lower limbs of an infant, particularly over the convexities and sparing the nappy-protected skin.

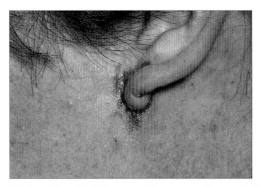

Plate 1.7   Child's ear. The crease beneath the ear is a favourite site for rubbing in atopic patient's, often creating superficial fissuring. In this patient secondary infection is just beginning.

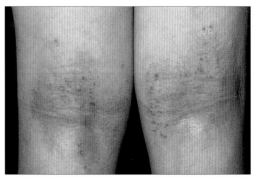

Plate 1.8   Popliteal fossae. The limb folds are a classical site for atopic eczema in childhood. This may be because particulate allergens, for example house dust mite and animal danders, stick and are concentrated in these damp flexures.

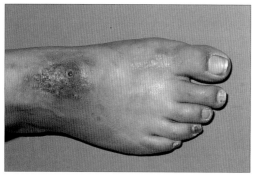

Plate 1.9 Patch of lichenification over the front of the ankle — the site that is most easily rubbed against the opposing calf. Note: in this Indian patient the marked post-inflammatory hyperpigmentation.

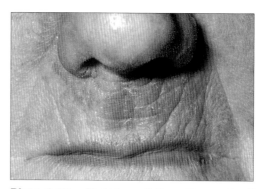

Plate 1.10 Rubbing of the skin under the nose can cause marked lichenification — a classical physical sign in atopic eczema.

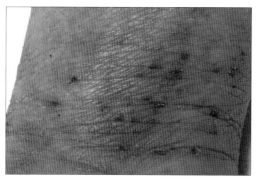

Plate 1.11 Typical lichenified and excoriated skin of atopic eczema of the wrist. This accessible area is a site of frequent rubbing and scratching.

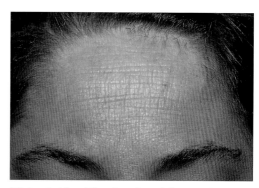

Plate 1.12 The forehead is another area easily rubbed or scratched. Usually the back of the hand is rubbed across the forehead causing the lichenification seen in this patient.

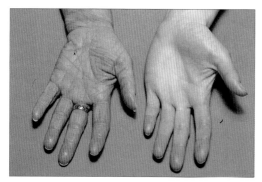

Plate 1.13 The hand on the left is atopic and has been much used for rubbing. This results in epidemal thickening, throwing into relief the normally invisible skin creases — so-called hyperlinearity of the palms. Note the normal hand on the right for comparison.

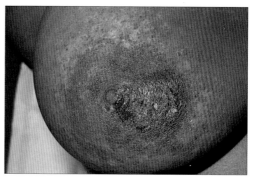

Plate 1.14 Nipples are a common site for atopic eczema in both males and females. In this case there is much lichenification and considerable post-inflammatory hyperpigmentation.

7

inantly on all **accessible** areas: often the nappy and shoe areas remain spared (Plates 1.4 and 1.6). If the eyelids are rubbed, the skin can thicken to form extra skin-folds under the eyes: the Dennie–Morgan folds (Plate 1.5). Another characteristic physical sign can be fissuring beneath the ear lobes (Plate 1.7), caused by repetitive and violent rubbing. Similar behaviour causes damage to the skin over the wrists below the cuffs (Plate 1.11), and to the neck above the collar-line. Areas of skin thickening (**lichenification**) can be seen at the top of the ankles, where they have been rubbed against the opposing calves.

Over four years of age, the limb flexures are usually most affected, with characteristic oozing and bleeding from excoriated and lichenified skin. This localisation may reflect the tendency of allergenic particles to stick to the damp, occluded surfaces, rather than to the exposed and drier convexities of the limbs (Plate 1.8).

If atopic skin disease persists into the teens and adulthood, it can leave the flexures for the surfaces of the limbs, as well as the trunk, neck, face, scalp, hands and feet (Fig 1.9). Occupational and personal habits influence the distribution. Any area exposed to regular friction, scratching or picking will show the characteristic excoriated lichenification of chronic atopic skin disease.

Exposure to environmental factors will make the face, neck and hands particularly vulnerable to acute exacerbations. These begin with local inflammation, dryness and intense pruritus, and progress to the chronic condition if they are not treated promptly and effectively.

In pigmented skin the regular trauma and inflammation of chronic atopic eczema is associated with damage to the dermo-epidermal junction, where the melanocytes lie. Released pigment granules are then collected by dermal macrophages. This process leads to a brownish dermal tattoo, **post-inflammatory pigmentation**, giving the skin an 'unwashed' or 'dirty' appearance (Plates 1.9 and 1.14).

Dryness of skin is a cardinal finding in atopic skin disease, and represents subclinical eczema. It may be complained of as a symptom, and recognised as a sign: there is a loss of the natural sheen or **bloom** of the skin. In its place the surface is dry, and can be scaly and fissured. Such skin is sensitive, and will smart when exposed to soap and water.

Fig 1.9 Common Sites of Chronic Eczema in Childhood and Adulthood

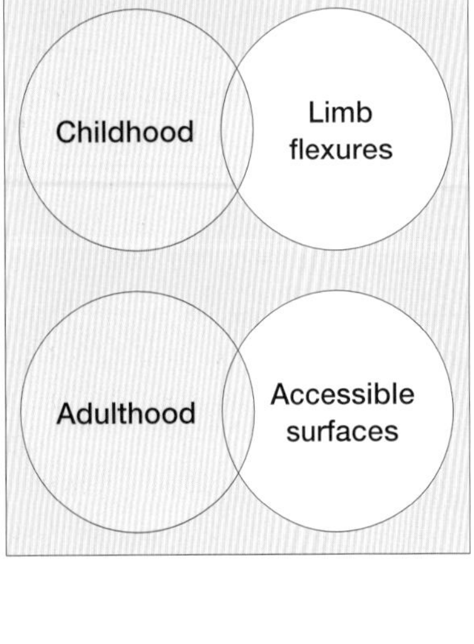

Childhood — Limb flexures

Adulthood — Accessible surfaces

Fig 1.10 Diagnostic Criteria for Atopic Eczema

Must have:	An itchy skin condition

Plus three of the following:

1. History of itchy rash
   Infants: on cheeks
   Others: skin creases (elbows, knees, front of ankles or under neck)

2. History of asthma or hay fever (under 4: family history in first degree relative)

3. Generalised dry skin in the past year

4. Visible eczema
   Under 4: over convexities (cheeks, forehead, outer arms)
   Over 4: in creases (as in 1 above)

5. Onset in first two years of life

The diagnostic criteria for atopic eczema as agreed by a working party of the Royal College of Physicians, London in 1995 are given in Fig 1.10.

Laboratory investigations

While there is no exclusive test to corroborate the diagnosis, 90% of patients will have a raised IgE level. This is the immunoglobulin that is associated with allergies. Total IgE level, and RAST tests for IgE to specific allergens can be helpful in planning management. These levels correlate well with reactions to skin-prick tests with the same substance (read at 20 minutes).

Histology

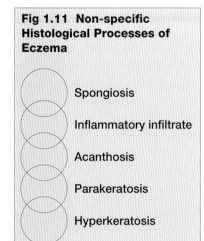

Fig 1.11 Non-specific Histological Processes of Eczema

Spongiosis

Inflammatory infiltrate

Acanthosis

Parakeratosis

Hyperkeratosis

The histology of atopic skin disease is similar to that of all forms of eczema (Fig 1.11) (see also p. 14, Plates 2.1–2.3). In the acute stage there are characteristic large epidermal vesicles, but all stages of the disease show similar epidermal **spongiosis**, and infiltration with lymphocytes. The inflammatory process in the dermis includes vasodilation and extravasation of blood cells into the upper dermis. The presence of eosinophils amongst the infiltrate can be seen in all types of eczema.

The basal layer of the epidermis is overactive and the even dermal pegs of a normal dermo-epidermal junction are replaced by great variations in thickness of the epidermis. Lichenification in chronic eczema shows histologically as a gross thickening (**acanthosis**) of the

9

epidermis with a piling up of cells, superficial nucleated keratinocytes (**parakeratosis**) and thickening of the horny layer (**hyperkeratosis**). Such changes are however non-specific and can be seen in any skin thickened by mechanical trauma, as in **lichen simplex chronicus** and **nodular prurigo**.

1.3 Atopic Skin Disease and The Environment

While the atopic state gives the individual a propensity to allergy, this is a much more obvious issue in asthma and hay fever than in atopic dermatitis. In the former conditions the causative role of specific allergy is fairly easy to demonstrate.

In atopic eczema there has been much discussion about possible causative allergens. Considerable research on large numbers of patients has failed to yield convincing evidence that **diet** is a significant causative factor for the majority. It is certainly sensible to consider a trial of dietary manipulation when a particular history is strongly suggestive. For adults this is rare, but occasionally it is helpful in infancy. Professional dietetic advice and supervision is always recommended.

The epidemiological evidence of an increase in the prevalence of atopic eczema in the urbanized western environment is however noteworthy. The typical modern home has tight-fitting doors and windows, all firmly closed against draughts and intruders. It is often double glazed and chimneys are closed, trapping human and **pet dander**, particularly in bedding and fitted carpets. Central heating then creates an ideal environment for an exponential rise in the population of the **house dust mite**. Knowledge of this, together with the results of specific immunological investigations of individual patients, and the experience of clinical improvement following appropriate environmental measures, has established the relevance for many patients of such interventions.

These include mite impervious covers for bedding, hard floors in place of fitted carpets, and more efficient vacuum cleaners. Further advice is available by contacting the agencies listed in Appendix 8.

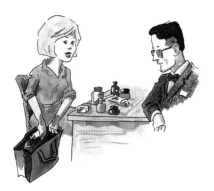

2

CONVENTIONAL TREATMENT

2.1 Emollient therapy

Introduction

The complex functions of the skin can be compromised by variations in skin structure. Drying of the skin, either through normal processes or disease, represents the most common such phenomenon. The vulnerability of dry skin includes susceptibility to heat and further water loss, infections and allergy, and through itch, general damage caused by rubbing and scratching (Fig 2.1). As the skin dries, it becomes relatively brittle, and easily cracks. Surface movement causes shearing forces both within the epidermis, and between the epidermis and dermis. These forces would normally be accommodated by healthy skin, but can have disastrous effects when the skin is dry. Emollient therapy for dry skin is therefore important for both moisturising **and** lubricating, enabling a return to healthy flexibility, resilience and strength.

Genetic factors

There is a wide variation in the characteristics of skin, regardless of disease. One of the most significant of these variations is in dryness. A general dryness of the skin can be an expression of multifactorial genetic inheritance that is not linked to atopy. Some patients with atopy will have such constitutionally dry skin (**xerosis**), but this is not necessarily the case. Moreover, constitutional dryness of the skin, with or without atopy, does not necessarily manifest itself throughout life. After adolescence a previously dry skin can become essentially normal, though for some individuals dryness of the skin will remain a characteristic throughout life. Otherwise constitutional dryness only manifests itself under certain

Fig 2.1 The Vulnerabilities of Dry Skin

Water and heat loss
Infections and hypersensitivities
Mechanical damage

11

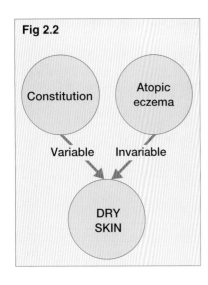

Fig 2.2

Constitution

Atopic eczema

Variable   Invariable

DRY SKIN

conditions — it can depend for example on weather, climate and season (Fig 2.2).

Cultural values

The cosmetic, preservative and therapeutic effects of emollient applications to the skin were evidently appreciated by the ancient Egyptians, Greeks and Romans. It seems likely that people of all cultures today similarly understand the importance of moisturisers for enhancing, protecting, and preserving the skin. Commercial considerations have led to the successful promotion of a multitude of preparations claiming near miraculous properties. Cultural and cosmetic considerations are necessary for treating skin disease successfully (Fig 2.3). The user-unfriendliness of some emollients is associated with poor compliance, despite the possibility that, at least for diseased skin, 'the more oily the preparation the better the effect'.

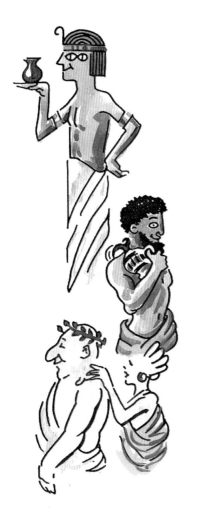

Fig 2.3 Emollients

Cheap can be better
than expensive
●
Build on current
cultural values
●
Ensure cosmetic
acceptability

Histology, physiology and the effects of disease

Three histological features are of interest in understanding the relevance of emollient therapy for dry skin: the intracellular water-holding characteristics of the keratinocyte, the lipid layers between the epidermal cells, and the desmosomes (Fig 2.4).

Natural moisturising factors (NMFs)

These complex proteins, carbohydrates and salts within the internal matrix of the epidermal cells, are found in greatest concentration in the cells closest to the surface of the skin. Pathological processes including atopic skin

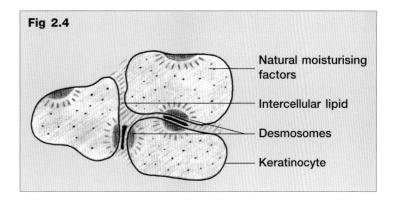

Fig 2.4

Natural moisturising factors

Intercellular lipid

Desmosomes

Keratinocyte

disease, that disturb the normal process of regeneration and maturation of epidermal cells, seem to be associated also with abnormalities in the concentration and distribution of the intracellular NMFs, with resultant reduced water-holding characteristics for the epidermis.

Intercellular lipid

There are between normal and healthy keratinocytes well-ordered layers of lipid. In contrast to the NMFs, these layers are found throughout the epidermis. While they provide both intercellular adhesion and flexibility, their properties include an essential insulation against otherwise excessive intercellular water permeation, and hence evaporation from the surface. Atopic skin disease causes an increased and more-or-less unregulated basal cell division, leading not only to smaller superficial keratinocytes — this itself increases water permeation — but also to deficiencies in the more superficial lipid layers. These deficiencies, which can evidently be considerably exaggerated by the injudicious use of water in combination with soaps and detergents, contribute significantly to excessive water loss, and drying of the skin. It is also possible that seasonal changes in intercellular lipid composition help explain the increase in atopic skin disease in winter.

Desmosomes

It is relevant also to consider the contribution of the desmosomes to the integrity of the healthy epidermis. These intercellular tying structures provide extra adhesion and therefore strength, and under normal circumstances they go through gradual enzymatic breakdown as the keratinocytes migrate to the surface, finally allowing the

13

Plate 2.1 Normal skin (H&E ×46). The regular cellular architecture of the epidermis provides both strength and flexibility. The epidermis is of even thickness, in contrast to that seen in chronic eczema.

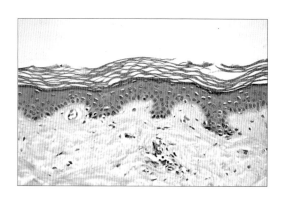

Plate 2.2 Acute eczema (H&E ×46). The regular epidermal layers are interupted by areas of spongiosis, associated with structural weakness. Infiltrating inflammatory cells cause characteristic redness, and itch.

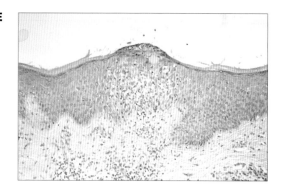

Plate 2.3 Chronic eczema (H&E ×46). The epidermis is greatly thickened, with an accentuated stratum corneum. The epidermal thickness varies considerably, with disturbed cellular architecture caused by increased cell division.

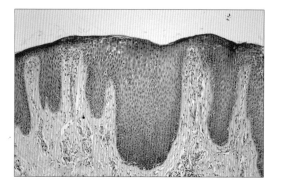

shedding of cells from the surface. With the abnormalities that develop in the surface lipid layers in atopic skin disease, there is a failure in the enzymatic breakdown of desmosomes. This phenomenon contributes to the characteristic thickening of the horny layer seen in atopic dermatitis. Here emollient therapy is important in providing lubrication and therefore flexibility to the damaged skin, which is otherwise vulnerable to further damage by scratching and rubbing (see Plates 2.1–2.3).

The skin as a semi-permeable membrane

As well as disease processes like atopic eczema, it is important to note that any increase in evaporation generates an acceleration in cell division in the lower parts of the epidermis, leading to disorganisation in the normal maturation process of the keratinocyte, and the abnormalities in histology and therefore physiology outlined above. Furthermore, not only does water balance on either side of the skin depend on the histology, physiology and certain morbid states of the skin, it also depends on variations in both the external surrounding environment, and in the internal environment of the body (Fig 2.5).

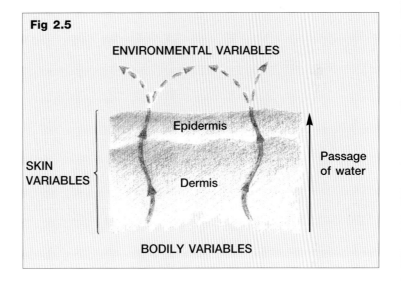

Fig 2.5

ENVIRONMENTAL VARIABLES

SKIN VARIABLES

Epidermis

Dermis

Passage of water

BODILY VARIABLES

External factors (Fig 2.6)

The relative humidity of the surrounding air, together with air movement and ventilation, links the effects of several phenomena that are notorious in their effects on the health of skin. Outside our modern buildings and modes of transport, season, climate and weather play on the equilibrium. Just like an old piano, in the cold, and therefore dry, air of the winter, the skin can go 'out of tune' if remedial action is not taken. Away from the fresh air, indoors in modern homes and offices, or travelling in modern cars, trains and planes, the unfriendly effects of central heating and air conditioning need to be allowed for. The skin thus requires the same consideration as the ancient books in our libraries and antique furniture in our museums.

Fig 2.6 Environmental Variables

- Climate, season and weather

- Air conditioning

- Central heating

- Relative humidity

15

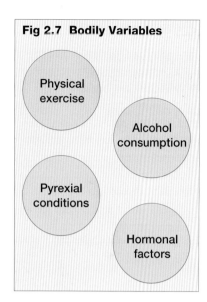

Fig 2.7 Bodily Variables

Physical exercise

Alcohol consumption

Pyrexial conditions

Hormonal factors

Internal factors (Fig 2.7)

Inside the body, on the other side of the skin, internal changes are significant for the water-balancing act that the skin is asked to accomplish. Thus, physical exercise requiring heat loss, and the hormonal changes of the menstrual cycle may exacerbate atopic dermatitis by accelerating water loss through the skin. Similar effects can result from excessive alcohol intake, toxic pyrexial conditions and any other state leading to dehydration of the body, especially when the water-holding ability of the skin is already compromised by existing atopic skin disease.

How do emollients work?

A filter analogy

The effect on water passage from skin to the surrounding air of an intervening layer of emollient depends on the amount of water arriving on one side of the emollient layer, the surrounding air conditions, and certain fixed characteristics of the emollient. Two important characteristics are the water-holding capacity of the moisturiser, and its own water permeability. Once the emollient is saturated, water will be held back in the skin when the rate of arrival of water from beneath exceeds the rate at which water can permeate through the emollient to the surface for evaporation.

Fig 2.8 Key Messages

On normal skin emollients lubricate rather than moisturise

•

On diseased skin emollients both lubricate and moisturise

Normal and diseased skin

Under normal conditions relatively little water passes through the epidermis. Emollient use on healthy skin may function more as a lubricant than a moisturiser, as the water passage through normal epidermis fails both to exceed the water-holding and the water permeation characteristics of the emollient. As explained above, diseased skin allows trans-epidermal water permeation at a greater rate. Under these conditions both epidermal moisturising and lubrication become significant (Fig 2.8).

Emollients, physiology and histopathology (Fig 2.9)

Experimental deficiencies in NMF concentration in the superficial epidermis have suggested the possibility that the effectiveness of emollients might be improved if they contained NMFs. An added factor, such as urea, might

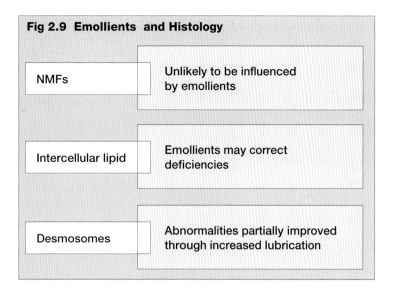

Fig 2.9 Emollients and Histology

NMFs	Unlikely to be influenced by emollients
Intercellular lipid	Emollients may correct deficiencies
Desmosomes	Abnormalities partially improved through increased lubrication

penetrate otherwise ailing cells and restore at least some water-binding capacity. However, no evidence has been forthcoming that this can be achieved. Incorporating NMFs into emollients does not seem to improve their effectiveness.

As explained above, deficiencies in the epidermal intercellular lipid layers seen in eczema not only lead to poor intercellular adhesion and epidermal flexibility, but also to decreased water-holding capacity and increased water permeation. The moisturising effect of an emollient is thought to be achieved partly through the direct occlusive effect described above, but the possibility remains that externally applied lipid can also be incorporated into the deficient layers.

The abnormalities in desmosome function seen in eczema are not directly corrected by moisturisation. Rather, emollient therapy may restore some of the lost flexibility caused by the failure of desmosome breakdown. Whether added lipid can influence desmosome function directly is not known.

The important clinical effectiveness of emollient therapy can therefore only be partly explained by current knowledge. Our ability to understand how emollients slow water permeation and evaporation, and provide lubrication in eczema remains relatively rudimentary and speculative.

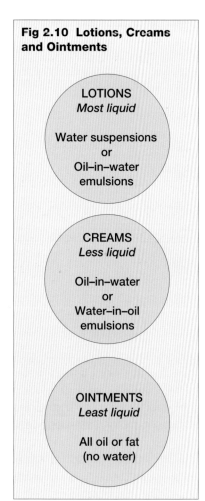

Fig 2.10 Lotions, Creams and Ointments

LOTIONS
Most liquid

Water suspensions
or
Oil–in–water
emulsions

CREAMS
Less liquid

Oil–in–water
or
Water–in–oil
emulsions

OINTMENTS
Least liquid

All oil or fat
(no water)

Fig 2.11 Oils and Fats in Emollients

Mineral, e.g. petroleum jelly

Animal, e.g. lanolin

Vegetable, e.g. arachis oil

Synthetic, e.g. cetomacrogol

Types of emollient

Lotions, creams and ointments (Fig 2.10)

Formularies such as the British National Formulary provide basic introductory information on the chemical properties and constituents of the vast array of emollients available. Ointments are thicker and less easy to use than creams, and creams are thicker than lotions.

Lotions can be suspensions, or emulsions. Suspensions, or shake lotions, contain insoluble powders and have little use in treating atopic skin disease. Lotions that are oil-in-water mixtures need an emulsifying agent to maintain the mixture. Additional active substances can be dissolved in either phase. Oil-in-water lotions are also rarely useful in atopic skin disease as their moisturising effect is short-lived and their lubricating function is minimal. They are however cooling in their effect, and may be useful in treating hairy skin.

Creams may be either oil-in-water or water-in-oil emulsions. The type is determined by the emulsifying agent used. Once applied most of the water evaporates, though some is absorbed by the superficial epidermis. The most relevant effect is the film of oil left on the skin surface. The oils used in creams may be synthetic, or may be mineral, animal or vegetable in origin. As with lotions, added ingredients can be dissolved in either phase of a particular cream.

Ointments are the most greasy of these three preparations. As they are more occlusive than creams, they are particularly suitable for chronic, dry lesions. Ointments do not contain water, but added constituents such as macrogol can make them easier to rinse off the skin. Various types of paraffin or petroleum jelly provide the bases of most popular ointments, but oils and fats from animal and vegetable sources are also used, as are those of synthetic origin (Fig 2.11).

Additives

Additional substances in lotions, creams and ointments are introduced with a variety of intentions. These include improving their user-friendliness, adding preservative and anti-inflammatory functions, and providing additional penetrating and hydrating qualities to the topical treatment.

These various effects need to be balanced against possible side-effects, in particular hypersensitivity.

Formularies such as the British National Formulary list commonly used additives according to the likelihood of skin sensitisation. There are more additives in lotions and creams than in ointments.

What emollients are available ?

A selection of emollients for use in atopic skin disease is given in Appendix 4. Emollients can be prescribed, or can be bought over-the-counter. They are usually ready made, but they can be made up according to a favourite recipe.

The most relevant principle is that **patient preference** is more important than **professional prescription** (Fig 2.12). With the approach described in this manual hopefully the patient becomes thoroughly aware of the rationale for effective emollient use, and chooses the best preparations for themselves. A trial pack of a variety of products can help considerably.

Mechanical topical treatments: pastes, bandages, wraps and hydrocolloid dressings (Fig 2.13)

A paste is a stiff preparation with a high content of finely powdered solids such as zinc oxide or starch, suspended in an ointment. Pastes can be useful as emollients, and also provide protection against environmental factors, but pastes are less occlusive than ointments. Pastes can be used as a vehicle for traditional antiseptic and anti-inflammatory remedies such as coal tar.

Bandages and wraps take mechanical protection a stage further than pastes, providing similar additional functions with easier application to larger areas of chronic atopic skin disease. Bandaging or wraps over topical steroids give quick relief, while preventing further scratching and rubbing damaging the fragile skin. Such treatment in day and in-patient care probably has a significant secondary psychological function in emphasising the need to give skin care a high priority.

The use of various mechanical aids in the management of atopic skin disease in both children and adults was greatly reduced by the introduction of topical steroids. It is likely now that the introduction of behaviour modification strategies into dermatological practice will reduce the use of mechanical techniques even further. The use of cotton gloves and body suits for infants is evidently unreliable protection against rubbing and scratching: the

Fig 2.12 Key Message

Emollient Choice:

Patient preference

is more important than

Professional prescription

Fig 2.13 Mechanical Topical Treatments

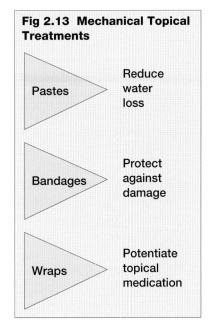

Pastes — Reduce water loss

Bandages — Protect against damage

Wraps — Potentiate topical medication

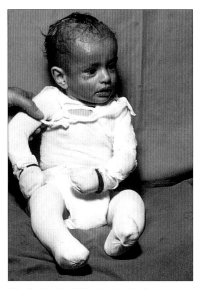

Plate 2.4 Whole body 'wraps' are often used for treatment of atopic dermatitis but scratching can easily occur through such dressings.

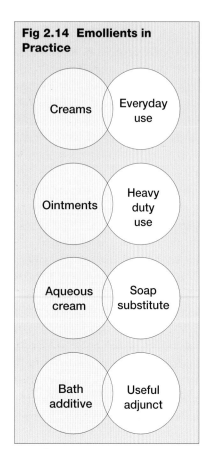

Fig 2.14 Emollients in Practice

Creams	Everyday use
Ointments	Heavy duty use
Aqueous cream	Soap substitute
Bath additive	Useful adjunct

layer of cotton can if anything provide an **aid** to effective rubbing and the creation of lichenification (Plate 2.4).

Amongst mechanical dressings an exception seems to be the hydrocolloid dressings. These semipermeable occlusive and adherent dressings can be useful in managing relatively circumscribed areas of chronic atopic skin disease. Used in conjunction with one application of topical steroid for each seven days of occlusion, such dressings provide treatment at all three levels of the vicious circle of chronic eczema (p. 61).

Emollient use in practice

What to recommend (Fig 2.14)

The general principles considered above help to explain all types of emollient therapy, but each can have its own particular usefulness. Clinical effectiveness depends partly on compliance, itself being determined by practical and cosmetic considerations. The most popular moisturisers are creams rather than ointments, and at any one moment immediately after a fresh application, a cream will be as effective as an ointment. To maintain emollient effect however, clinical experience suggests creams need more frequent application, especially at the beginning of treatment, while ointments are particularly useful in situations where the skin is most at risk of drying and damage by external factors. Aqueous cream in particular is useful as a substitute for soap. The cream is wiped on and used as a lubricant for gentle massage of the skin to be cleaned — vigorous rubbing is unnecessary and unhelpful — **before** being washed off in still or running water (Plates 2.5 and 2.6). For bathing and showering a number of preparations are mentioned in Appendix 4. Water contact is otherwise evidently unfriendly for eczematous skin. Simultaneous exposure to an emollient when bathing leaves the skin more flexible and comfortable on drying. The use of an additional layer of emollient after a warm bath is popular with many patients, the idea being that 'following a good soak' the moisturiser will prevent evaporation as the skin cools.

How, and when to use (Fig 2.15)

It is important to explain the practical tips that are given to the patient for emollient therapy (p. 65). There is no evidence for there being any advantage in applying a

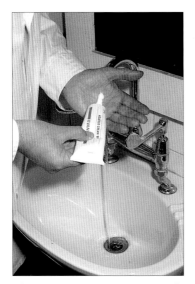

Plate 2.5 Aqueous cream. A tube should be kept by each sink so that it is easily available for use instead of soap. It should be very gently massaged on the skin **before** wetting the hands ...

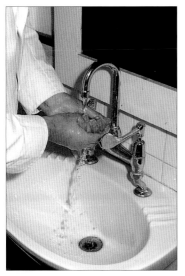

Plate 2.6 ... and then rinsed off.

Fig 2.15 The Hows and Whys of Emollient Use	
THINLY	Emollients prevent water loss, rather than add water to the skin
GENTLY	Dry, and eczematous skin is brittle and fragile
QUICKLY	Application should be easy and not time consuming
FREQUENTLY	Emollients should prevent drying rather than treat dryness

moisturiser thickly. Prevention of water loss, and not heat loss, is the object of the exercise. The water that will moisturise the skin comes largely from the body fluids below rather than from the applied cream, and therefore the thinnest possible application is preferable. Not only will this be effective, but it will be more cosmetically acceptable — if the emollient is opaque on application, it will become translucent more rapidly when only a small amount is used.

The structural characteristics of both dry, and eczematous skin, including brittle fragility and lack of normal flexibility, dictate the relevance of gentle wiping on of a moisturiser, and argue strongly against the common advice that the emollient should be **rubbed** into the skin. Such rough treatment is known by many patients to be equivalent to scratching, and is sometimes indulged in for that reason alone. Not only is rubbing unnecessary, it is contraindicated — it is a damaging process, and for some patients it **provokes** a significant itching reaction that then tempts an even more damaging scratching episode. The advice that topical applications should be accomplished **quickly** and **without fuss** aims similarly at avoiding unnecessary manipulation and therefore stimulation of the treated skin. It is useful to ask the patient at consultation to demonstrate how they apply their moisturiser. Almost invariably the cream is applied overvigorously and with much massage and rubbing. It can then be explained that this is inappropriate and counterproductive. The correct method can be easily demonstrated, and it will be seen immediately to be quicker and therefore easier. Frequent use, to achieve prevention rather than treatment of dry skin, becomes then a more feasible proposition.

21

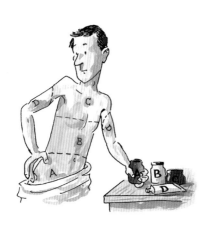

Different areas and different needs

Some areas will need more frequent treatment than others, depending on absence or presence of active disease, and the part of the body involved. Exposed areas, such as the head, neck and hands need the most frequent treatment.

Particular areas of the body are not served well by standard emollient preparations. The scalp, and the ear are such examples: suggestions for appropriate emollient therapy are given in Appendix 4.

Convenient amounts and the availability of emollient (Fig 2.16)

One practical aspect of emollient use that should not be overlooked when considering the importance of the frequency of use, is the convenient **availability** of the preparation. Understandably the large amounts that are often needed over time dictate bulk prescribing, usually in 500g dispensers. **Pump dispensers** are preferable to open tubs, to prevent the reservoir of emollient becoming a source of infection. Such containers are often kept at home in the bathroom. They do not lend themselves to being easily transported.

As emollients need to be available throughout the day, in different parts of the house and garden, in the car, at school or college or at work, thought needs to be given to ensuring that the patient does not get into practical difficulties. Smaller tubes of a particular preparation should be available; the pharmacist may be asked to supply small empty plastic containers to use, or the patient may discover the usefulness of empty 35mm photographic film containers.

Continuous versus discontinuous use

Although for a few patients it will be necessary to use emollients continuously, despite effective treatment of atopic skin disease, for many the result of such treatment allows for emollients to be discontinued. It is arguably preferable for moisturisers not to be used in a ritualistic fashion, but rather strictly **as required.** As is explained later (p. 79), in the follow-up phase of treatment it is continuous **vigilance** that is required. This attitude is more likely to be associated with appropriate proactive intervention, not only through the recognition that emollients are needed, but also by the early recognition of the clinical features of relapse in atopic eczema. Then

Fig 2.16 Key Messages

Large containers of moisturiser can become reservoirs of infection

•

Small amounts of emollient should be readily available throughout the day

active treatment can be started sooner rather than later, with better results (p. 81).

Emollients with topical steroids

All topical steroids need to be delivered to the skin in an emollient vehicle, usually a cream or an ointment. This may make the use of an emollient strictly unnecessary at the same time as using a topical steroid on the areas of the diseased skin being treated. However invariably when topical steroids are being used on diseased skin, potentially dry but not diseased skin needs emollient therapy, and this will be applied both at the same time that the topical steroids are applied, and at other times as necessary to prevent the skin from drying. We find it best practice to advise that when they are used together the topical steroid is applied first, directly to the eczema, and the emollient is then wiped on over both the steroid and over the skin needing only moisturiser. Thus the emollient can be described as a temporary semi-occlusive dressing over the steroid. This sequence may fit also with the observation made sometimes by patients that topical steroid therapy can be relatively astringent. It seems the skin needs more frequent moisturising when topical steroids are being used, especially when they are particularly potent.

It has been suggested that topical steroids are more likely to be effective when the skin has been 'rehydrated' with an emollient. If emollient therapy is provided for the skin on a regular and consistent basis, preventing the skin from drying rather than treating dry skin, steroids will always be applied to skin that has not dried — and the application of the emollient **after** the topical steroid can be seen then to have no particular disadvantage, while having the advantage of providing the temporary occlusive effect that is thought to increase topical steroid effectiveness as well as adding a further general protective layer against environmental hazards.

2.2 Topical Steroids

History

Compared with the use of emollients, topical steroids have been a very recent introduction. While emollients have some use on healthy skin, the use of topical steroids is restricted to the treatment of inflammatory skin disease.

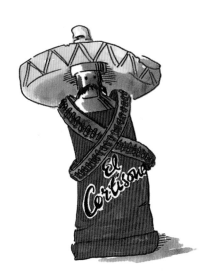

The first synthetic glucocorticosteroid, hydrocortisone, was created in the early 1950s, and the effect of topical hydrocortisone on the management of inflammatory skin disease was immediate and revolutionary. Since then progress has been fast. By manipulating the cortisone molecule it proved possible to increase very considerably the anti-inflammatory potency. Unfortunately every increase in potency brought with it an increased tendency to cause thinning of the skin. This side-effect on both epidermis and dermis gives the skin an aged and wrinkled appearance, and makes it particularly vulnerable to trauma. Research continues to strive to dissociate side-effects from anti-inflammatory effect, but so far without convincing success.

Pharmacology

Corticosteroids are normal circulating hormones, and **all cells** in the body have steroid receptors. When supra-physiological doses of natural hydrocortisone, or one of the more potent synthetic analogues (e.g. betamethasone valerate) reach these receptors, dramatic changes occur. These effects are chiefly inhibitory: less protein synthesis, less secretion of products, less cell division, and less migration of cells. Hence the anti-inflammatory effect derives from (a) reduction in lymphokines secreted by lymphocytes, and (b) reduced activity of eosinophils, neutrophils, and basophils.

Topical steroids are conventionally divided into four main potency groups (p. 157). In the United Kingdom and many other countries only hydrocortisone acetate preparations (1% or less) can be obtained over-the-counter without prescription.

Close examination of the molecular configuration of the steroids found in each potency group reveals few if any clues as to the link between chemical structure and therapeutic potential. The development of this particular part of the pharmacopoeia has been largely empirical. Changes in the side chain of a particular molecule, e.g. hydrocortisone acetate to hydrocortisone 17-butyrate can bring significant changes in potency. For this reason it is considered safer in prescribing to use proprietary rather than approved names.

Although 'dilution' of a particular active steroid molecule in its cream or ointment vehicle may seem at first sight to reduce the **potency** of a particular preparation,

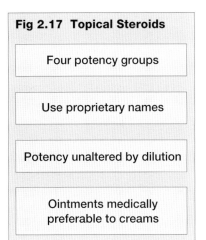

Fig 2.17 Topical Steroids

Four potency groups

Use proprietary names

Potency unaltered by dilution

Ointments medically preferable to creams

this is not the case. Such dilution serves only to reduce the **dose** of steroid per unit volume of any given preparation. However, use of a **cream** or **ointment** vehicle may be relevant regarding potency, as ointments provide a semi-occlusive effect that can increase potency. Furthermore the bio-availability of the topical steroid can be enhanced by certain additional constituents, e.g. propylene glycol, and keratolytic agents like salicylic acid and urea. Hydrocortisone acetate 1% moves from the 'mildly potent' group of topical steroids to the group termed 'moderately potent' with the addition of urea to the preparation.

The cream and ointment vehicles used to deliver steroids to the skin have similarities to those used as emollients, but additional constituents are required to dissolve the otherwise insoluble steroid molecule. Although one well known topical steroid vehicle is also available as a separate emollient, vehicles are not generally available separately. While a **patient's preference** for a cream needs to be acknowledged to ensure optimal compliance, the potentially sensitising additives in creams sometimes make ointments **medically preferable** (Fig 2.17).

Therapeutic effects

Epidermis (Fig 2.18)
Topical glucocorticosteroids cause a reduction in the rate of epidermal basal cell division. As has been described, the increased rate of epidermal proliferation (acanthosis) seen in lichenified atopic skin disease leads to the main structural and functional abnormalities of the condition. As cell division is reduced, so the epidermal architecture and physiology return to normal.

Dermis (Fig 2.18)
The steroid action in the dermis blocks the release of a variety of inflammatory substances from both white and mast cells, as well as blocking the effects of released substances (interstitial oedema, attraction of further neutrophils, and the generation of pruritus). The direct effect of glucocorticosteroid on the white blood cells of the inflammatory process is one of reduction in number, activity and secretion. Whether the observed local vasoconstriction associated with steroid action contributes to the therapeutic effect remains uncertain, but it is a curious fact that there is a direct correlation

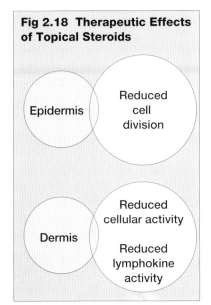

Fig 2.18 Therapeutic Effects of Topical Steroids

Epidermis — Reduced cell division

Dermis — Reduced cellular activity / Reduced lymphokine activity

25

between anti-inflammatory potency of a given corticosteroid molecule and its vasoconstrictor activity.

Two stages in steroid effect (Fig 2.19)

As will be discussed later (pp. 66–67) one of the common mistakes in using topical steroids is **stopping too soon.** Once the skin 'looks good' topical steroid therapy is discontinued. This fails to take account of the two-phase characteristic of topical steroid therapeutic effect. The healing progress under the influence of topical steroids occurs from 'outside–in'. When the epidermis first appears to the eye intact and healed again, there are still hidden beneath the epidermis clusters of active inflammatory cells in the dermis. If steroid therapy is discontinued at this point, the inflammatory process can take hold again and the epidermis will break down with an early relapse of the eczema. It is therefore necessary to continue steroid treatment for a further period after epidermal or 'cosmetic' healing has been achieved, in order to obtain the second phase of dermal or 'histological' healing.

In early eczema relapses, both stages in topical steroid effect can be achieved in days. In chronic eczema, using **The Combined Approach**, each stage takes two or three weeks, though natural healing processes not requiring steroid therapy will continue for a further two or three months.

Side-effects

Types, and relevant factors

The side-effects caused by topical steroids are both **local** and **systemic**, and the chance of them complicating treatment, together with the severity of the effects, depends on four factors: the potency of the steroid used, the amount that is used (i.e. the extent of the body treated), the length of the treatment period, and the site being treated.

Local side-effects

There can be a reduction in thickness of both epidermis and dermis (Plates 2.7 and 2.8). In the epidermis, whether thinning occurs through a reduction in the volume of cells, or in the number of cells continues to be debated. In the dermis there is evidence that topical steroids inhibit collagen formation with resultant

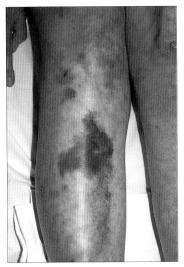

Plate 2.7 Steroid atrophy.
Steroids can cause epidermal and dermal thinning with easy bruisability here caused by over-zealous used of grade I topical steroid ointment.

Fig 2.20 Local Side-effects of Topical Steroids

Epidermal thinning →	Ulceration
Reduced dermal collagen →	Telangiectasia, purpura and ageing
Reduced dermal elasticity →	Striae
Increased sebaceous activity →	Acne
Hair follicles stimulated →	Hirsutism
Reduced immune response →	Infections exacerbated, and disguised

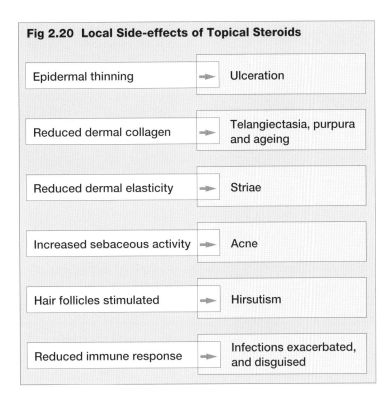

structural weakness. The lessened support for blood vessels explains the easy development of **purpura** as a local complication.

Such early changes may be reversible. Later atrophic changes associated with longer term treatment are not (Fig 2.20). These include the development of **striae** through elastic tissue damage (Plate 2.9), and skin **ulceration.** On the face especially, **telangiectasia** rarely spontaneously remits, but can be treated (p. 41).

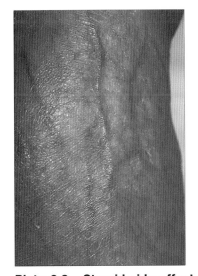

Plate 2.8 Steroid side-effect.
Marked dermal atrophy revealing veins usually hidden by a dermis of normal thickness.

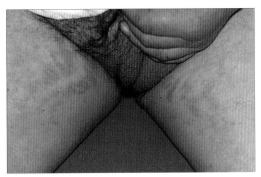

Plate 2.9 Striae. These striae in this young man's groin were induced by the injudicious use of a grade II topical steroid in this occluded site.

27

Plate 2.10   Steroid acne. A curiously confined grouped of acne lesions with open and closed comedones induced by over-enthusiastic use of potent topical steroids.

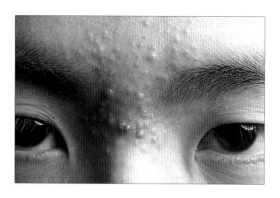

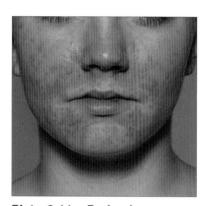

Plate 2.11   Perioral dermatitis. Note the scores of tiny sore red 'bumps' scattered over the lower face with striking sparing just around the vermillion of the lips. This side-effect of grade I and II topical corticosteroids is virtually never seen with grade IV steroids and rarely with grade III. It responds well to oral tetracycline.

Acne, or **rosacea** can be local, potentially reversible side-effects on the face for some individuals (Plate 2.10). **Perioral dermatitis** is a similar condition around the mouth, usually of younger people, and particularly women (Plate 2.11). Increased sebaceous activity can lead also to other acneform eruptions. Hirsutism is an occasional side-effect, caused by stimulation of steroid dependent hair follicles. Bacterial, fungal and viral infections may be exacerbated, or disguised.

Although potent topical steroid use can cause skin lightening by inhibiting melanocyte function, the normally increased melanocyte activity induced by sun exposure is also inhibited by the inflammatory process itself. This is a reversible phenomenon.

The risk of local side-effects

Many studies of local side-effects, both experimental on healthy skin, and clinical on diseased skin (not always atopic eczema) have been published in recent years. Although certain overall observations are possible from a review of this research, it remains difficult to generate from these investigations any firm guiding principles. As in all fields of investigation, there are difficulties in comparing different studies. There are differences in terminology and definition, inherent difficulties in assessment, differences in study design and problems in comparing the effects on healthy skin with those seen in disease.

That experimental studies of topical steroid effects show more evidence of skin thinning than is demonstrated by clinical studies is striking. Unfortunately it is not always clear if **atrophy** is being used as a general term including reversible epidermal thinning, or whether it is being reserved for the irreversible changes outlined above. Moreover most studies only report on these important

---

Fig 2.21 Key Message

With topical steroids ...

Side-effects come from inappropriate use

Good effects come from appropriate use

---

effects — other local side-effects, and central systemic effects are not often considered. Evidently in clinical studies the relative absence of the particular side-effects being studied must in part be related to the presence of the disease process, and the behavioural complications associated with it. Thus, as skin is thinned by a topical steroid, it is thickened by the characteristic rubbing and scratching associated with atopic skin disease. The latter phenomenon needs to be allowed for when considering experimental studies using healthy skin.

What we can conclude at present is that local side-effects are associated with injudicious and inappropriate use of topical steroids. The risk of skin atrophy from topical steroid use cannot be ignored. However, when used correctly only benefits accrue (Fig 2.21). The Combined Approach described in this manual both sets out the protocol for the best use of topical steroids, and depends on their **good effects for good results.**

Systemic side-effects

Not only is it convenient and otherwise rational to treat skin disease with steroids by topical application, this route clearly helps avoid systemic side-effects. Even so, a particularly important hazard of topical steroid use is the possibility of absorbed glucocorticosteroids in the circulation leading to a depression of the hypothalamo-pituitary-adrenocortical axis. This leads to a reduction in naturally circulating corticosteroids, demonstrable by estimating the 9 a.m. blood cortisol level. In extreme and fortunately rare cases it is possible with topical steroids to induce iatrogenic Cushing's syndrome, followed by Addison's disease on withdrawal.

Although regular small amounts of prescribed systemic steroids can induce other systemic side-effects in adults (p. 33) these are not reported systemic side-effects of topical steroids. In children any possible systemic effects need to be distinguished from effects on development caused by eczema and asthma themselves (p. 32).

Topical steroids in clinical practice

Attitudes to topical steroids

Our clinical experience using the programme described in this manual is that problems with topical steroids can be expected when they are used inappropriately and without due regard to all aspects of the condition being treated.

Side-effects in long-standing atopic skin disease can be avoided if the aims of treatment rather than the fear of side-effects dictate the behaviour of both doctor and patient. Hence the relevance of the discussion with every patient of the nature of atopy (p. 58) as an unavoidable constitutional vulnerability, compared with atopic skin disease as an eminently treatable condition. A vigorous treatment approach reduces the severity, length and frequency of relapse in atopic eczema, and eliminates chronicity for the great majority of patients (p. 83, Fig 4.37).

The Combined Approach

In practice we emphasise that it is essential that topical steroids are not used in isolation. For an acute relapse their use is combined with appropriate emollient therapy, and in the management of chronic eczema topical steroid and emollient therapy **must** be complemented by simultaneous attention to eliminating self-damaging behaviour.

Steroid use on different parts

In the same way that topical steroids come in four potencies, the natural sensitivity of skin to topical steroids varies according to part treated. While the stronger steroids are sometimes required for the hands, feet and scalp, the weakest may be appropriate for the face, and genital area. Other parts are intermediate in sensitivity, though care should be taken with the thin skin on the inside of the thighs and upper arms. In disease, lichenification can make otherwise sensitive skin relatively resistant to topical steroids. Then even on the face the strongest steroids may be required, under close supervision and as part of a planned treatment programme. Apart from different strengths, some areas such as the scalp, and ears may pose practical problems. Suggestions for what to use are given in Appendix 4.

Strengths, frequencies and amounts (Fig 2.22)

It is invaluable to create with each patient a clear and strict schedule for them to follow. Simplicity will make this easier. There are disadvantages in providing a range of steroids in different strengths to use in sequence, and one or possibly two should be sufficient if varying the frequency of application is part of the programme. Most topical steroids are used on a twice daily basis. Some new preparations are used once daily. While there may

Fig 2.22 Key Message

*Ensure appropriate topical steroid use by **educating the patient** and by providing a **clear treatment schedule***

be no advantage in increasing this recommended frequency, reducing the frequency can be appropriate in the later stages of histological healing (pp. 67 and 80). Thus a therapeutic effect can then be expected using a topical steroid once on alternative days. The frequency of use on different parts, such as the scalp, should follow general principles adapted by particular practical considerations.

The amount of topical steroid used on a part on one particular application should only be sufficient to 'shine the skin'. It is unnecessary and counterproductive to rub in the cream or ointment. 'Wiping on' is the optimal method. Use of the '**only a shine is necessary**' principle will always ensure that only appropriate amounts are used. If the topical steroid is applied before the emollient, the 'shining technique' is easy to achieve.

When deciding on the amount of topical steroid to prescribe on a particular occasion, apart from the patient's own practical experience, two over-riding and important principles must be borne in mind. Over-generous prescribing, combined with a planned programme based on **total healing** as the aim, is preferable to under-prescribing, with attendant risks of inadequate treatment. Once the aim of treatment has been achieved, there seem to be no disadvantages in having a half-empty tube remaining. Secondly, should the patient come close to running out, they should know how to get a fresh supply, and understand the importance of doing so.

The length of the active treatment programme
The Combined Approach aims to establish topical treatment as an intermittent rather than continuous process. Taking account of the four weeks required for a normal basal cell to progress to shedded squame, it is not surprising that it may require four to six weeks topical treatment to achieve first **cosmetic**, then **histological** healing when treating chronic eczema. An acute relapse can however be successfully managed in as many days, using the same two-phase model. Premature cessation of treatment in either chronic eczema or acute relapse will be followed by further acute disease sooner rather than later. The effect of The Combined Approach is to reduce the total amount of topical steroid used, with consequent reduction in any likelihood of local or systemic side-effects.

Topical steroids for children, infants and babies
Understandably the concern over both local and systemic side-effects increases with the youth of the patient. Although very young patients have skin that may be very responsive to topical steroids, there is also the attendant fear of increased risk of side-effects. Such concern is generated by common clinical experience.

If however all aspects of The Combined Approach are taken into account the same principles in topical steroid use are applicable whatever the age of the patient. As with all patients, close monitoring of the healing process is relevant. Overall, less rather than more topical steroid use will result from The Combined Approach in children, just as with adults. Inadequate treatment of children, infants and babies leads to chronic disability. When this is profound, the effect on development and growth can be as alarming as the retardation caused by systemic side-effects.

There is little evidence that systemic effects of topical steroids stunt growth in children. More important may be the stunting effect of regularly interrupted sleep in chronic eczema, as growth hormone is usually released in sleep. When lack of sleep complicates long-standing atopic skin disease through itch and scratching, there is a related reduction in growth hormone secretion. If the child also suffers from severe asthma, hypoxia is an additional factor in stunting growth.

2.3 Other Treatments

Antihistamines

Topical antihistamines should not be used as there is considerable risk of sensitisation.

Oral antihistamine preparations are frequently prescribed but the results can be disappointing, despite the theoretical logic behind their use. In childhood a sedating antihistamine at night can be helpful, though it may be the sedative rather than the antihistaminic effect that is important. Promethazine and trimeprazine are often used.

For adults, hydroxyzine or its non-sedating derivative cetirizine may be prescribed. That much scratching in chronic eczema is habitual and not provoked by itch may help explain the unsatisfactory results of antihistamine treatment. See Fig 2.23.

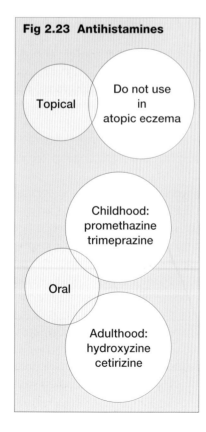

Fig 2.23 Antihistamines

Topical

Do not use in atopic eczema

Childhood: promethazine trimeprazine

Oral

Adulthood: hydroxyzine cetirizine

Counter-irritants and topical anti-pruritics

Apart from systemic antihistamines, topical moisturisers and corticosteroid creams and ointments, there is occasional place for traditional remedies in reducing pruritus in atopic skin disease. Counter-irritation of the skin with 0.5% menthol in aqueous cream, and the use of preparations containing lauromacrogols (p. 155), can be useful soothing additions to a particular treatment programme. Oatmeal bath preparations can have similar effects.

Evening primrose oil

Evidence for the therapeutic value of evening primrose oil in atopic skin disease remains inconclusive. Based on evidence that some children with atopic dermatitis show reduced levels of the essential fatty acid gamma linoleic acid (GLA) in their blood, the provision of supplements in the form of evening primrose oil is thought by some to improve the clinical symptoms of atopic eczema. As a **natural** treatment, it is often popular. To assess its effectiveness for an individual patient adequate doses need to be given for three months. If no benefit is then noted, it is unlikely to be helpful.

Sometimes taken by adults as well as given to children, GLA may have a potential to manifest undiagnosed temporal lobe epilepsy. This can occur when epileptogenic drugs such as phenothiazines are also being prescribed (Fig 2.24).

Fig 2.24 Evening Primrose Oil

- A popular complementary remedy

- Uncertain effectiveness in atopic eczema

- Discontinue if unhelpful after thorough trial

- Beware epileptogenic property

Systemic steroids

Few clinicians regard systemic steroids as a sensible long-term option for the treatment of atopic skin disease. Side-effects emerge sooner or later, including growth retardation, diabetes mellitus, osteoporosis, hypertension and the exacerbation of infection. The dramatically beneficial effects seen when they are used in the management of urticaria, angio-oedema, asthma and allergic rhinitis are much less obvious in atopic eczema. This may be explained by the time required for the resolution of skin lichenification and dermal inflammation. Locally applied corticosteroids have a much superior therapeutic ratio (effect/side-effect) compared with systemic steroids. In addition, with eczema of differing severity at

Fig 2.25 Systemic Steroid Therapy

- Short-term gains not dramatic

- Long-term treatment contra-indicated

- Occasionally useful
  - tetracosactrin 1 mg IM
  - triamcinolone 40 mg IM

Fig 2.26 Cyclosporin A

Useful in transplant surgery

Disappointing in other chronic inflammatory conditions

Dramatic acute benefit in atopic skin disease

Side-effects limit long-term use

Fig 2.27 Azathioprine

Useful adjunct in managing other chronic inflammatory conditions

Temporary suppressing effect atopic eczema

Long-term use limited by risk of side–effects

different sites, the range of topical steroids available at varying potencies allows for better fine-tuning of treatment.

However, the occasional use of a single injection of glucocorticosteroid, or synthetic corticotrophin can be an expedient intervention, within an overall plan of treatment (Fig 2.25).

Cyclosporin A

Introduced as an immunosuppressant drug, it is used to inhibit the lymphocyte-mediated rejection of transplanted organs, including kidneys, heart and bone marrow. Although its anti-inflammatory effect in rheumatoid arthritis and auto-immune diseases has been disappointing, it has dramatically successful effects in atopic eczema. Itch is suppressed in days (Fig 2.26).

The beneficial effects only continue while the drug is taken. As it also causes dose-dependent kidney damage and hypertension in the majority of patients treated, it is a remedy held in reserve for only the most severe and refractory patients.

Azathioprine

This drug inhibits cell division and is useful as an immunosuppressant in the treatment of rheumatoid arthritis and auto-immune conditions. It is most often useful as an adjunct to the more rapidly effective systemic steroids, enabling their dosage to be more quickly curtailed (Fig 2.27).

As with cyclosporin A, azathioprine has only a temporary suppressing effect on atopic dermatitis. Because of the possibility of malignant disease with long-term use, it is also reserved for the most treatment-resistant cases.

Ultra-violet light phototherapy (UVB and PUVA)

Patients and parents often but not always notice a gratifying improvement in atopic eczema after a sunny beach holiday. Such improvement may have a multifactorial basis. Day-time exertion gives deeper sleep, relaxation and diversion both reduce scratching, and sea-bathing may have an antiseptic effect. While an overdosage of sun-rays damages the skin and causes blistering and peeling, a lower dosage clears the skin of the more

Fig 2.28 Phototherapy

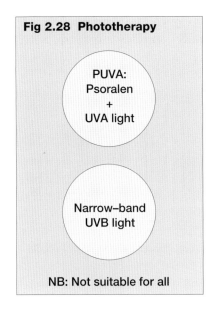

PUVA:
Psoralen
+
UVA light

Narrow–band
UVB light

NB: Not suitable for all

vulnerable cells associated with the immune response: lymphocytes, macrophages, neutrophils and eosinophils. Hence there is a reduction in the inflammatory process, and an improvement in atopic skin disease. Therapeutic UV lights aims to simulate the benefits of sunshine. The UVA lights used in tanning parlours, gyms and health clubs exert however little benefit in eczema. UVA combined with **psoralens** either orally or in a bath (PUVA treatment) can be helpful, as can narrow-band UVB treatment. The treatment produces a temporary remission in selected patients who can tolerate photo-therapy (Fig 2.28).

Provided only in specialist centres, the disadvantages of phototherapy include premature photo-ageing and skin malignancy, as well as both expense and incon-venience.

Chinese herbs

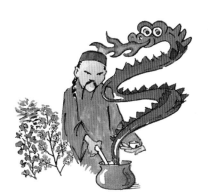

Teas made by prolonged boiling of combinations of selected dried plant material have been used for centuries by traditional Chinese healers (Fig 2.29). The success of such remedies for atopic skin disease has been investi-gated by western dermatologists in recent years and the beneficial effect of the treatment has been confirmed, with acceptable short-term toxicity margins. Liver function tests should however be carried out, both before and after treatment.

The decoctions are however unpalatable, although encapsulated forms are being developed. During long-term therapy, toxicity, especially in children, remains a worrying factor. The only non-steroidal western drug to similarly suppress atopic eczema is Cyclosporin A, and the late emergence of malignancy is its recognised occasional side-effect.

Hypnotherapy

Stage hypnotherapists have led to hypnosis being discred-ited in the public and medical eye as a valid medical treat-ment. However, in skilful hands, the technique has been reported to improve atopic eczema in the long and short term, in adults and children. Several sessions are required and the techniques for inducing adult trance need consid-erable modification for use in children. Suggestions are aimed at curtailing scratching, decreasing sleeplessness

Fig 2.29 Chinese Herbs

An effective
traditional
remedy

Unpalatable,
and potentially
toxic

35

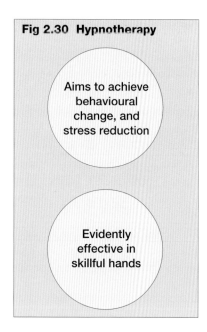

Fig 2.30 Hypnotherapy

Aims to achieve behavioural change, and stress reduction

Evidently effective in skillful hands

and minimising ambient anxiety. The technique would appear to have few side-effects but, like habit reversal, currently suffers from a severe limitation of availability (Fig 2.30).

Future avenues

Genetic research may be able to further localise the genes which confer the potential to atopic allergies. However, it would currently seem unlikely that genetic engineering could reduce this immunological response without prejudicing other important defence mechanisms.

Less toxic analogues of Cyclosporin A could be valuable suppressive medicines. Elucidation of the active principles in Chinese herbs might open many new therapeutic doors, and allow better toxicological evaluation.

A more immediate and achievable prospect would be an easy and safe way of controlling the vastly increased population of house dust mites in the modern house. The new comfortable and effective covers for bedding are a crude but excellent first step forwards minimizing exposure to the 20th century midden within the home.

2.4 Complications During Conventional Treatment

Treatment of atopic eczema with emollients and topical steroids can be frustrated by two complications in particular: **hypersensitivity reactions** and **infections.**

Hypersensitivity reactions

Hypersensitivity can occur as contact reactions to both emollients and topical steroids. There is both inflammation and an unexpected lack of response to treatment. The inflammation may only show itself when topical steroid treatment is discontinued (Fig 2.31).

Emollient hypersensitivity
Reactions to moisturisers are relatively rare, and given the wide range of preparations and products available, it is invariably possible to find alternatives when necessary. Hypersensitivity is usually due to an added preservative or perfume. Amongst the oils and fats used in emollients, only lanolin (sheep sebum) is notorious as a sensitiser.

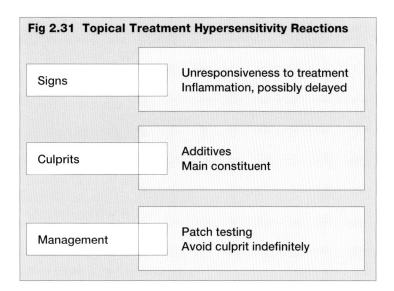

Fig 2.31 Topical Treatment Hypersensitivity Reactions

Signs	Unresponsiveness to treatment Inflammation, possibly delayed
Culprits	Additives Main constituent
Management	Patch testing Avoid culprit indefinitely

Topical steroid hypersensitivity

Hypersensitivity can occur as a reaction to ingredients in the vehicle, or to the steroid molecule itself. Reactions to the steroid molecule seem to be rare, but should always be considered possible.

Management

Hypersensitivities to topical treatments need to be investigated by patch testing in specialist units (Plate 2.12). Once identified the culprit needs to be avoided indefinitely, as desensitisation is not effective.

Fig 2.32 Key Messages

Infections

Atopy: impaired immune response

•

Bacteria multiply in dry scaly skin

•

Creams and ointments block follicles

Infections

Atopic eczema is susceptible to secondary bacterial, fungal and viral infections. Various factors contribute to this vulnerability. Thus the disturbed histology causes defective barrier function; commensal micro-organisms such as *Staphylococcus aureus* can multiply enormously in the dry and scaly skin. Furthermore, the necessary use of creams and ointments allows hair follicles to become blocked with oils and fats, contributing to the pathogenesis of folliculitis. Finally, atopy itself as a constitutional state can carry with it a vulnerability to infection through deficiencies in immune response (Fig 2.32).

Bacterial infections (Fig 2.33)

Staphylococcus aureus is the most common bacterial pathogen in atopic eczema. The inflammation that

37

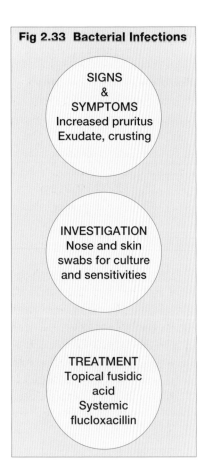

Fig 2.33 Bacterial Infections

SIGNS
&
SYMPTOMS
Increased pruritus
Exudate, crusting

INVESTIGATION
Nose and skin
swabs for culture
and sensitivities

TREATMENT
Topical fusidic
acid
Systemic
flucloxacillin

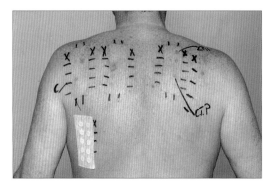

Plate 2.12   Delayed hypersensitivity investigated by patch testing. Allergens are applied, dispersed in white soft paraffin in aluminium cups, applied in sets of 10 on non-allergic tape (left lower back). They are read at 48 hours. In this patient several positives are easily visible. Interpretation of patch test reactions needs much experience to differentiate true allergy from irritant reactions. True delayed cutaneous hypersensitivity is lifelong and positive patch tests are repeatable. In practice in atopic eczema patch tests are chiefly useful for identifying and hence eliminating secondary hypersensitivities, e.g. to medicaments, nickel and preservatives.

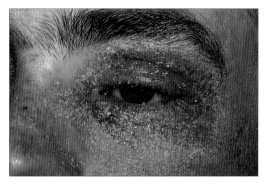

Plate 2.13   Bacterial infection. When an area of lichenification becomes wet and sticky, as around this eye, secondary infection has probably occurred. The most usual organism is *Staphylococcus aureus*.

Plate 2.14   Bacterial infection. Infection deep in the pores of an eczematous area causes inflamed folliculitis as seen in this child's ankle. The organisms are streptococci or staphylococci. Such infection is favoured by the use of topic corticosteroids, occlusion and tar.

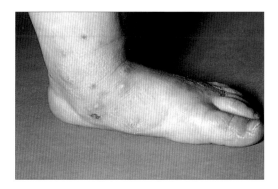

accompanies an infection can be associated with an increase in pruritus, together with a weeping exudate and crusting (Plates 2.13 and 2.14). Swabs from the nose and the skin should be taken for culture and sensitivities. Antibiotic treatment can be local and systemic. A combined antibiotic and steroid cream can be used, though some antibiotics are notorious for causing hyper-sensitivity reactions when used topically. Fusidic acid is often a preferred local treatment. Flucloxacillin is a useful systemic antibiotic. Otherwise mupirocin (Bactroban) ointment and triclosan (in Ster–Zac concentrate) bath additive can be useful.

Fungal infections (Fig 2.34)

Although atopic skin disease may increase the risk of fungal infections, such complications are unusual. A dermatophyte infection, such as *Trichophyton rubrum*, can sometimes explain the failure of atopic eczema on the hands to respond to conventional treatment. The topical steroid can obscure the diagnosis, and skin scrapings for microscopy and culture may be necessary. Both topical, e.g. imidazole, and systemic treatments, e.g. terbinafine, are effective. The choice depends on the severity of the condition.

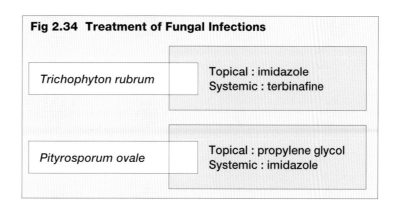

Fig 2.34 Treatment of Fungal Infections

Trichophyton rubrum	Topical : imidazole Systemic : terbinafine
Pityrosporum ovale	Topical : propylene glycol Systemic : imidazole

Pityrosporum ovale (Malassezia furfur) is a yeast that normally colonises the skin, and occasionally complicates atopic eczema with pityrosporum folliculitis, or pityriasis versicolor. It can also complicate atopic skin disease with a hypersensitivity reaction. The folliculitis affects the back and the chest, sometimes the face and neck, with an intensely itchy and pustular rash (Plate 2.15). Pityriasis versicolor produces depigmented patches with a branny

39

Plate 2.15 Fungus infection in an atopic patient treated with topical steroids, giving the so-called tinea occulta pattern with fugus driven deep into the follicles.

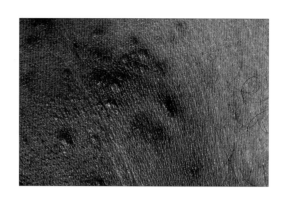

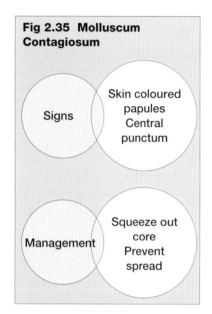

Fig 2.35 Molluscum Contagiosum

Signs — Skin coloured papules Central punctum

Management — Squeeze out core Prevent spread

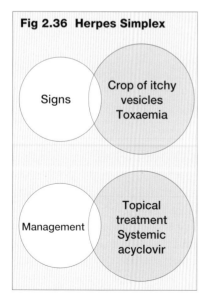

Fig 2.36 Herpes Simplex

Signs — Crop of itchy vesicles Toxaemia

Management — Topical treatment Systemic acyclovir

scaling over the upper trunk especially. Topical, or systemic imidazoles, or topical propylene glycol preparations are used in treatment but this needs to be persistent to get good results.

Viral Infections

Atopic individuals also have an increased susceptibility to viral infections, some of which can become serious.

Molluscum contagiosum (Fig 2.35) is common among children with atopic eczema. It is spread by body contact. Skin coloured papules with a central punctum or umbilicus are found particularly in the flexures, but can appear on any part of the body. The distribution may reflect the mode of contagion. Secondary bacterial infection may complicate the condition. Treatment techniques are various, and include squeezing out the cheesy core from each lesion using forceps, after application of a local anaesthetic. Common sense measures help prevent spread to others.

Herpes simplex (Fig 2.36) sometimes causes serious problems (Plate 2.16). Eczema herpeticum can be localized, but when severe and widespread the condition is life-threatening. Characteristic sharply circumscribed itchy vesicles appear, especially on the face. Secondary bacterial infection is common, together with lymphadenopathy, fever, headache and malaise.

Diagnosis can be confirmed by examination of the vesicular fluid with electron microscopy, by immunofluorescence, or by viral culture. Systemic treatment with acyclovir has improved dramatically the prognosis of the condition. Topical treatment includes diluted potassium permanganate compresses, and continuing topical steroid treatment. Any secondary bacterial infection will need appropriate treatment.

Plate 2.16 Eczema herpeticum. Sudden worsening of atopic dermatitis with sheets of tiny papules, which on close inspection show central dimples and perhaps vesicule formation, is the hallmark of herpes simplex spreading in eczema. This needs urgent systemic acyclovir, usually intravenously.

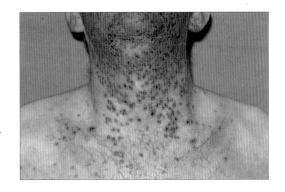

People who develop herpes labialis (cold sores) should avoid intimate contact with anyone with atopic skin disease.

2.5 Managing Local and Systemic Side-Effects of Steroid Therapy

The ethos of The Combined Approach to atopic skin disease is to **prevent the side-effects** of steroids. The behaviour modification technique of **habit reversal** (p. 43), and the educational emphasis of the approach aims to reduce dramatically the use of steroid treatment. This recognises that once side-effects of steroid treatment have become established, management can become very difficult.

Local side-effects

Epidermal thinning
This is reversible if the potency of the topical steroid can be reduced, or the treatment discontinued. It may be that for a short period topical treatment can be replaced by a systemic treatment (pp. 33–35) (Fig 2.37).

Dermal atrophy
There is no treatment for the loss of elastic tissue. Loss of collagen may be very gradually replaced, reducing the incidence of purpura. Telangiectasia can be treated with electrical hyfrecation, or laser treatment. Continuing treatment of atopic eczema can become very difficult. Further damage can only be prevented by minimising the use of further steroid treatment, topical or systemic.

Fig 2.37 Key Messages

When topical steroids cause local side-effects

- *Reduce potency*

- *Minimise use*

41

Acne, rosacea, perioral dermatitis and other steroid acneform eruptions

All these conditions require both review of and if possible reduction of the potency of the topical steroid being used, together with the prescription of a systemic antibiotic such as tetracycline, for several weeks.

Hirsutism

This unusual but distressing side-effect of steroid therapy is slowly reversible if the potency of the steroid treatment can be reduced, or the treatment discontinued.

Exacerbation or masking of skin infections

The possibility of such phenomena causing additional problems needs to be constantly considered, particularly when the treatment of atopic skin disease seems inexplicably ineffective. A high degree of suspicion will prompt an appropriate investigation, leading to the diagnosis and correct treatment.

Systemic side-effects

The management of the systemic side-effects of steroid therapy is beyond the scope of this manual. They are fortunately very rare, and the introduction of habit reversal and The Combined Approach should make such complications of the treatment of atopic eczema exceptionally rare in the future.

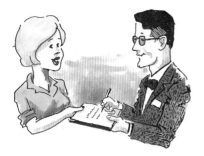

3
HABIT REVERSAL

3.1 Introduction

Habit reversal is a psychological method for treating disorders such as tics and nail biting, that can also be used to help patients with atopic skin disease to stop scratching. Although it is a behaviour modification technique based on principles of behavioural psychotherapy, habit reversal can also be seen to be a method based on common sense. It is not time consuming. Indeed as part of The Combined Approach, overall it is very cost-effective. One is not required to be a trained behaviour therapist to use the technique, but to achieve the best results it is necessary to use the full procedure. In the management of long-term atopic skin disease the effectiveness of habit reversal depends on it being offered **together with effective conventional treatment**.

3.2 An Earlier Application

The work in Uppsala, Sweden by Melin, Norén and their colleagues (1986, 1989, 1995) was based on the earlier work of Azrin and Nunn (1973) in the United States. They described habit reversal as a method for eliminating unwanted nervous habits and tics. A nervous habit was defined as a behaviour starting as a normal response to a physical injury. Through positive reinforcement the behaviour increases in frequency and becomes established as a habit with an automatic nature. As this occurs, there characteristically develops an associated lack of personal and social awareness. At the same time, the habit **generalises** — a variety of situations become potential precipitants of the response (Fig 3.1).

Azrin and Nunn described their work with 12 patients aged 5–64 years, with complaints ranging from shoulder

---

Fig 3.1 Development of a Nervous Habit

- Normal initial specific response

- Increased frequency by positive reinforcement

- Behaviour becomes automatic

- Stimuli become more general

- Decreased personal and social awareness

43

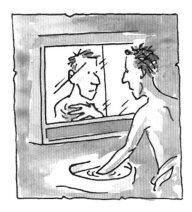

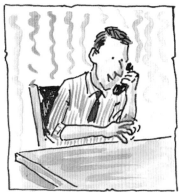

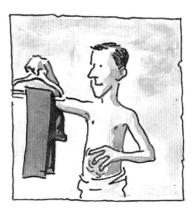

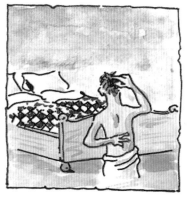

and head jerking and shaking, to eyelash plucking, finger-nail biting and thumb sucking. All were first involved in a week's recording of the frequency of their behaviour. This process was termed 'registration'. It was an integral part of the treatment programme, as the behaviour in question had to be made conscious before modification could be successful. Each patient then required a tailor-made new behaviour pattern which

(a) was opposite to the old habit,
(b) could be maintained for several minutes,
(c) was socially acceptable and compatible with normal activities, and
(d) strengthened the muscles antagonistic to those used in the old habit.

Those with head jerking and head shaking were instructed about isometric contraction of the neck muscles. For eyelash picking, thumb sucking and fingernail biting the advice was to grasp a suitable object until muscular tension could be subjectively detected in the arms.

Habit reversal reduced the undesired behaviours by at least 90% for all subjects after three weeks. A longer term follow-up showed excellent results for seven of the subjects. It was concluded that habit reversal could be an effective behavioural technique for patients of all ages and for both high and low frequencies of undesirable habitual behaviours.

3.3 Applications for Atopic Skin Disease — Research

Prior to the work done by Azrin and Nunn, the relationship between the histological appearance of long-standing atopic skin disease and rubbing and scratching had been clearly linked by experimental work using 'scratching machines': experiments with mechanical irritation on normal skin and patients with atopic skin disease produced similar histologic reactions, the main characteristics of which are identical to those seen in long-standing atopic skin disease (see Appendix 9 for References and Further Reading).

Could the habit reversal techniques of Azrin and Nunn be adapted therefore for the management of scratching behaviour in atopic eczema? Here the nervous habit is

scratching, which starts out as a normal, understandable behaviour in response to the feeling of **itch.** If scratching is thus provoked for a sufficient length of time, and increases in frequency, awareness is reduced and the behaviour becomes automatic. At the same time it links to circumstances, situations and activities over and above the original itching stimulus. In the skin the result is the lichenification of chronic eczema.

Thus in long-term atopic skin disease much scratching is **habitual**, whereas the scratching of acute eczema can be all in response to **itch**.

Melin and his colleagues in the earlier study (1986) arranged for patients to be taught habit reversal by two psychology students. After an initial period of registration of scratching frequency without treatment, the patients were divided into two groups. Both groups used topical hydrocortisone for four weeks, but only one group was instructed in habit reversal. Instead of scratching they learnt to grasp an object, or clench their fists.

Both groups improved, but the scratching frequency after four weeks was reduced by 90% in the habit reversal plus hydrocortisone group, against 60% in those using hydrocortisone alone. The eczema score showed an improvement of 70% using habit reversal compared with 30% without.

As these results seemed promising, the technique was developed. In contrast to nail-biting, scratching **can** be provoked by a physical stimulus: **itching**. If itch could be diminished at the same time by habit reversal, a more successful treatment might be expected.

Although scratching can provoke itch, part of the effect of scratching is to relieve itch. Experimentally pruritus in a particular dermatome can be diminished by pricking a needle into the skin of the same dermatome. Furthermore, some patients volunteer the knowledge that they can pinch, or press a nail into an itching area and experience relief. Some use the technique as a remedy for the discomfort caused by insect bites.

Based on these observations the later study (Norén and Melin, 1989) used

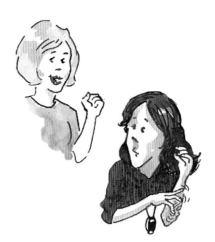

(a) clenching the fists and counting to 30 as an alternative to the **habit** of scratching, then
(b) pinching the skin where it was itching as an alternative to **itch-provoked** scratching

as the new, desirable behaviours to replace scratching in atopic eczema.

45

Forty-six patients with chronic atopic skin disease used hand-counters to 'register' their daily scratching frequency, and after one week they were randomly allocated to one of four groups. Two groups used topical hydrocortisone for four weeks, the other two used topical betamethasone-17-valerate for two weeks followed by hydrocortisone for two weeks. One group from each different topical steroid schedule were taught the new habit reversal procedure.

Reduction in scratching frequency and improvement in eczema score were statistically significant for the habit reversal patients, compared with those using topical steroids alone. It was important to note however no patients showed **complete** healing at four weeks, and use of a potent steroid for two weeks, followed by hydrocortisone for two weeks led to several examples of relapse.

Although scratching could be diminished by 90% in three days by habit reversal, healing then required longer periods of effective topical treatment.

3.4 Habit reversal in practice

The above research studies generated ideas that have since been modified and improved upon in continuing clinical practice. The programme initially consisted of two parts — registration, then active treatment. From the start integral to the treatment was an educational element using written material. Later it was realised that follow-up was very important (Fig 3.2).

Habit reversal is not usually involved at follow-up. Adequate topical treatment of subsequent relapses of atopic eczema, once the chronic syndrome has been successfully treated, is the essential intervention. The risk of the re-emergence of chronic eczema must always be guarded against however, largely by the patient being proactive and aware of how the syndrome develops.

More than anything, clinical experience has confirmed many times over the results of research: habit reversal offers the clinician a potent treatment opportunity in the management of atopic skin disease, but only when it is combined with adequate conventional topical treatment: it is not a treatment that stands on its own. Clinical practice has also highlighted how much more can be achieved by enabling the patient to manage their own condition. Changes in attitude are associated with improved prognosis. When difficulties in achieving a

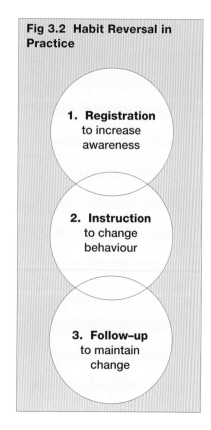

Fig 3.2 Habit Reversal in Practice

1. **Registration** to increase awareness

2. **Instruction** to change behaviour

3. **Follow–up** to maintain change

Fig 3.3 Characteristics of The Combined Approach

Pharmacological treatment enhanced by behavioural change

Treatment package adapted to individual requirements

Variety of cost–effective adaptations possible

satisfactory outcome occur, although biological factors may be relevant, the psychosocial issues reviewed in Chapter 4 can be of even more importance.

Behavioural treatments are therefore always more potent when assessment is able to take account of personality factors and relevant social influences. Insensitively delivered, 'off the peg' treatments are never as successful as those that can be tailored to the individual's needs. For the great majority of patients this attention to detail need not become time-consuming. The 'minimal effective dose' is of relevance in behaviour modification, as it is in physical medicine.

All the work that has led to the development of this manual has been done with individuals on a one-to-one basis. Other workers including Ehlers and her colleagues in Germany (1995) have successfully incorporated a habit reversal technique into a group approach. This clearly is of interest as a cost-effective adaptation. Behavioural treatments also lend themselves to self-help approaches, and it may be in the future that a self-help manual based on The Combined Approach will enable more patients to benefit from its effectiveness (Fig 3.3).

In recent years behavioural treatment programmes have been designed for use on personal computers. That some patients have asserted a preference for computers over seeing a health professional may be interpreted in various ways, but as a method of providing treatment for as many people as possible, the use of computer programmes may prove important in the future management of atopic skin disease.

3.5 Habit Reversal and the Very Young

Fig 3.4 Working with the Very Young

Habitual scratching starts early in life

Scratching develops an emotional significance

Success depends on parental involvement

Early intervention prevents chronicity

It is evident that some of the difficulties that adults have in their psychological adjustment to long-standing atopic skin disease may originate in childhood experiences: the earliest symptoms of atopic eczema often pre-date language acquisition. Scratching behaviour can clearly become a potent method of non-verbal communication between child and concerned parents. Many adults will admit that the emotional significance of their scratching goes back to a childhood need for support from significant others (Fig 3.4).

Habit reversal offers parents an approach to atopic eczema in their child that is not only effective as part of

47

The Combined Approach, but in being so effective may prevent future difficulties as the child grows up. The treatment approach for adults has been successfully adapted for children, as set out in Chapter 5. The younger the child, the more it is necessary to adapt the adult programme, but the principles can be applied in practice to patients of all ages.

Just as in adults, children present with 'itch scratching' and 'circumstance scratching'. Children as young as three years old can learn the 'pinch' technique described above, and benefit from active participation in their treatment. Probably the most important general rule with children is however the total avoidance of the **negative entreaty**,

'Stop scratching!'

which is replaced by a range of interventions that are characteristically positive and active. Clearly with children it is necessary to work with their parents, and in so doing the beliefs of the parents must be taken into account. This is particularly vital if either or both parents has suffered also with atopic eczema. If a parent has chronic atopic eczema themselves at the time a child is brought for treatment, serious consideration needs to be given to treating the parent first.

Fortunately treating very young patients can be considerably helped by their behaviour changing quickly. What can be achieved in two days with a child of two years can take weeks for an adult of 20. However the healing process in the skin still requires adequate treatment with emollients and topical steroids, and this process can last as long as it takes for adults (Fig 3.5).

Subsequently, as for adults, the follow-up programme for children requires continuing **vigilance** and prompt treatment of relapses. Habit reversal is not involved in such situations, providing the response is early and adequate. The debilitating syndrome of long-standing atopic skin disease can then be avoided altogether.

Fig 3.5 Key Messages

*Habit reversal is easy
to understand*

•

*Applies to the chronic
syndrome*

•

*A combined approach
is essential*

•

All ages can be treated

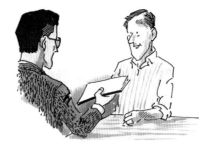

4

WORKING WITH ADULTS AND OLDER CHILDREN

4.1 Introduction

Age range

The approach described here for adults is appropriate also for teenagers and older primary school attenders, but it is necessary to involve the parents of younger patients. The programme for very young children is described separately in Chapter 5.

Themes and process

The structure of the programme naturally breaks down into a series of consultations, between which the patient assesses their condition at home, reads their handbook (Appendix 2), practises new behaviours, and discusses the programme with others both at home and elsewhere. The treatment process has several inter-related themes described below and highlighted in Fig 4.1.

Achievable goals
Discussion is needed on what can and what cannot be changed. While the constitutional state of atopy remains unavoidable, long-standing atopic skin disease is definitely avoidable for the great majority of patients. Complete remission of chronic disease, with only short-lived episodes of acute relapse, will become possible. Taking trouble in dealing with long-standing atopic skin disease is therefore a good investment of time and energy.

Fig 4.1 Key Messages

Activate involvement

•

Encourage realistic optimism

•

Promote biological understanding

•

Increase behavioural awareness

Attitudes

From the start there is a need to take into account existing assumptions and understanding of the illness, and throughout to use all opportunities to enable a shift from passive acceptance with pessimism, to active management with optimism.

Common sense and understanding

The programme is based on common sense and is easy to understand. The structure and function of normal skin is basic to the approach. The better the biology of skin is explained, the better the outcome.

Awareness

The approach requires a greater awareness of behaviour that is relevant to the condition of the skin. At both assessment and follow-up the implicit intention is to raise awareness, in order that self-management can be optimal.

Responsibility

Passive acceptance of a long-term illness is often encouraged by a particular professional to patient relationship, where the professional is seen as the 'expert'. It is useful constantly to try to move responsibility, together with expertise, from the professional to the patient. The patient then becomes their 'own expert'. Collaboration between the patient and therapist enables mutual understanding of the condition, and what is needed in treatment. Success depends on **the active involvement of the patient**, more than any other factor.

Measurement

In order to achieve awareness and then to follow progress in self-management, there needs to be an emphasis on clarifying **when**, **how often**, and **how much**. Such subjective assessments emphasise the patient being their own therapist, increasing the sense of personal responsibility for their own condition.

Structure: the consultations

To achieve worthwhile results it is necessary to see the patient several times over several weeks, with follow-up review at a few months, and perhaps a year. The number, length and frequency of these visits can be adapted to

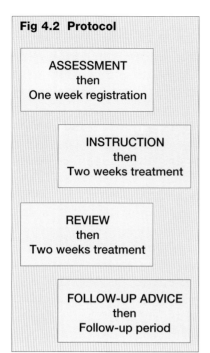

Fig 4.2 Protocol

ASSESSMENT
then
One week registration

INSTRUCTION
then
Two weeks treatment

REVIEW
then
Two weeks treatment

FOLLOW-UP ADVICE
then
Follow-up period

circumstances. What follows is only an illustration of the approach in practice (Fig 4.2). The themes of the process involved apply at each visit, with particular issues requiring review on more than one occasion, if change in attitude and successful self-management are to be accomplished. As major themes, Assessment, Treatment and Follow-up can be considered in sequence, though in practice these stages overlap and inter-relate considerably. The current protocols for visits at the Daniel Turner Department of Dermatology, Chelsea & Westminster Hospital are detailed in Appendix 1, though they are adapted frequently to suit particular patients, and varying circumstances.

Full and shorter versions

What follows is a complete account of all the techniques currently used. The protocols are only guidelines. It may well be that the 'minimal effective dose' will prove to be less than the full programme described. An approach where the essentials are explained and emphasised as logical can leave the individual to decide on how to proceed. Spending more rather than less time with our patients has however allowed us to gain a greater understanding of the otherwise 'secret world' of the atopic patient with skin disease. The impression gained is clear — the more time spent initially means less time spent later.

4.2 Assessment

Following referral the patient is seen at the Chelsea & Westminster Hospital for dermatological diagnosis before being referred on for The Combined Approach programme. Assessment for the programme begins with the second visit and continues through to the third visit, when overt treatment is introduced. In primary helath care, dermatological diagnosis and assessment for this programme can be simultaneous.

Explicit and implicit functions

Assessment is an obvious process to both therapist and patient — it clarifies the dermatological diagnosis, elucidates the history of illness, the current condition of the patient and the current treatment being used. A complete

51

assessment enables the making of an appropriate treatment plan that suits the needs of the individual patient. As these explicit purposes are worked through, implicit in assessment is a review of attitudes to illness and treatment, with the identification of any attitudes that are negative and therefore counterproductive. The fuller the assessment, the more clearly one can understand how the patient has used treatment to date. Early discussions in assessment set the scene for heightening awareness through registration of scratching behaviour, and for a complete analysis of all self-damaging behaviour.

As The Combined Approach programme is clearly different to other treatments the patient will have experienced, its main characteristics need introduction. It is particularly relevant to take into account that some patients with long-term atopic skin disease have tried many different treatments in the past, and have been very disappointed with the results. The patient can be advised that more time will be spent in consultations than they are used to, and attention will be especially paid to what happens between consultations. An early start is made towards achieving a positive and optimistic alliance with the patient. Occasionally doubts will be expressed about the rationale of the programme. If nevertheless the procedures involved can be accepted at face value and followed for long enough, changes in attitude follow.

History of presenting complaint

Overview

By going back to the first experience of eczema, even though it is often remembered second hand, as reported to the patient by parents, the way atopic dermatitis is often entangled with psychosocial factors can become an early topic for discussion. Especially when the illness begins in the first year of life, the involvement of the patient's mother in caring for the condition is relevant. It is worth asking whether the mother also had eczema, and if siblings suffered from the same condition. This information, together with the quality of the child–parent relationship, illuminates subsequent developments in the history and informs both management and estimation of prognosis. Occasionally patients with chronic atopic dermatitis in adult life are found to have established an emotional investment in keeping the condition, and the origins of this may be found in early childhood experiences.

This initial review also examines what is remembered, not only of the condition itself in the past — its distribution, severity, fluctuations, and treatment — but also its social and psychological repercussions. It is relevant to note the presence or absence of hayfever and asthma in childhood, as part of a discussion of the nature of atopy.

The course of illness until recently may include a period of complete recovery, followed by a recent relapse. It may be reported that the distribution of the condition changed significantly in adolescence.

Recent history

In order to clarify current experience and to compare with future progress, one should enquire about any recent fluctuations in the condition. This can be achieved by asking whether improvements and relapses last for days, weeks or months. Whether or not the condition ever completely clears, its effect on quality of life, and whether or not topical treatments are used continuously or intermittently all need consideration. This review is completed by asking about factors that seem to be associated with either worsening, or improving the condition.

Current state (Fig 4.3)

Using a simple range of 0–10, where 0 represents perfect skin and 10 represents the worst the skin condition has ever been, the patient can usually give their own score for their current state. This can be asked at each visit, to emphasise the importance of self-monitoring — and at the same time it is useful to ask how much of the current eczema is long-standing (months and years), compared with eczema that is relatively recent (up to two weeks) in origin. A subjective statement about which areas are **most** affected, and which areas are also involved, is noted. First mention of the relevance of **itch**, and **scratching** can be made at this point. Clarification of the difference between the two terms may be needed — itch is a **feeling**, and scratching is an **action**. The simple question:

'How much of your scratching comes from itch?'

usually prompts an important recognition that much scratching in long-term atopic dermatitis is not caused directly by itch. Circumstances, situations and activities are at least as important in provoking scratching once atopic eczema is chronic. This feature of scratching in

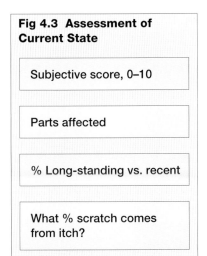

Fig 4.3 Assessment of Current State

Subjective score, 0–10

Parts affected

% Long-standing vs. recent

What % scratch comes from itch?

chronic eczema may never have been discussed before by the patient with a doctor or nurse. Sharing knowledge of scratching behaviour — how scratching sometimes 'connects eczema to the rest of life' allows for a joint appreciation of how complicated the situation has become.

Current treatment

Enquiry about current treatment, both prescribed and over-the-counter, illustrates well the difference between the explicit and implicit in assessment. It soon becomes clear, after several patients with long-term atopic skin disease have been assessed in this way, that many reach a point when use of conventional topical treatments becomes serendipitous and haphazard. Some fail to understand the difference between emollients and topical steroids, and even use the latter instead of the former. Differences in potency of topical steroid may be unknown or misunderstood. There can be a collection of medication accumulated at home which represents a pharmacist's Aladdin's cave. A tube of cream can be picked almost at random, based more on whim than any rational plan.

Wariness of topical steroids is a most significant issue. This needs early recognition as otherwise the worry over possible side-effects can be so strong as to undermine appropriate treatment significantly, despite careful and rational explanation. One way of exploring these attitudes is to enquire about the patient's experience of success when using topical steroids. A weaker steroid will sometimes have been chosen repetitively, despite failure to get good results. Discussing this experience makes the relevance of using steroids at effective strengths self-evident.

This part of assessment sets the scene for much of what will follow in the programme. The importance of education and careful explanation, both spoken and written, becomes evident. And the relevance of a written treatment plan and a record of treatment to be completed by the patient also becomes clear.

Behavioural analysis

With the topic of itch and scratch in atopic eczema already introduced, a focus on scratching can now be developed. The first part of **behavioural analysis** can be introduced at the end of the first visit. This sets the scene for the first homework assignment: **registration** of scratching frequency (p. 61). An analysis of the undesirable, to-be-changed behaviour follows a simple A–B–C

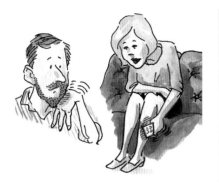

Fig 4.4 The ABC of Behavioural Analysis

Antecedents
   Situations, Circumstances and Activities associated with behaviour

Behaviour
   The behaviour itself – forms and frequencies

Consequences
   The physical, emotional and social results of the behaviour

---

Fig 4.5 Key Messages

Scratching is an objective behaviour

•

Itching is a subjective experience

Fig 4.6 Six Methods of Scratching

1. Nails, including picking

2. Rubbing skin on skin

3. Rubbing through cloth

4. Rubbing against object

5. Use of an instrument

6. Involving someone else

---

format of Antecedents, Behaviour, and Consequences (Fig 4.4). The enquiry serves to draw attention to and clarify the behaviours that need modification.

Antecedents. Questioning can take the patient through a 'typical day', from waking to sleeping again, and asking for each activity, situation and circumstance: *'Do you scratch then?'*, or *'When do you scratch?'*, and *'When do you never scratch?'*. Here there is a further opportunity to differentiate between scratching and itching, as it is scratching **behaviour** more than itching **experience** that is the focus for the analysis (Fig 4.5).

Particular patterns for the individual will emerge, illustrating issues that become relevant in planning treatment. Thus a behavioural characteristic for many adults who go out to work, is the scratching done on first returning home in the evening. For this there will need to be particular strategies devised as part of their **behavioural prescription** (p. 69).

Behaviour is detailed by asking about the methods of scratching employed (Fig 4.6). The seemingly infinite number of techniques possible, and the inventiveness of some individuals will quickly become clear (Plate 4.1). Questioning can open up otherwise intimate personal experience, and will demonstrate to the patient the therapist's interest and knowledge of self-damaging behaviours, preparing the ground favourably for the introduction of behaviour modification. The discussion of scratching method is placed in our protocol **after** registration, as the latter procedure increases awareness of self-damaging behaviour. Initial discussion of such behaviour can itself achieve this however, and can be effective therefore if introduced *before* registration. The

55

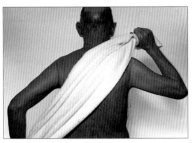

Plate 4.1   Scratching. Patients often use domestic events such as towelling after bathing to have 'a good scratch'. Many other domestic objects are used for scratching, e.g. hairbrushes, combs, furniture, even a partner's stubble!

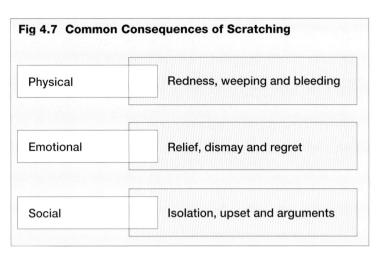

Fig 4.7   Common Consequences of Scratching

Physical		Redness, weeping and bleeding
Emotional		Relief, dismay and regret
Social		Isolation, upset and arguments

advantage of doing this is to make clear what behaviours will 'count' as scratching for *registration*.

Consequences are usefully divided into those that are (a) physical, (b) emotional, and (c) social. (Fig 4.7). Questioning can include: *'After vigorous scratching, how does your skin look and feel?'*, *'How do you then feel in yourself?'*, and *'What effect does all this have on those closest to you?'*.

Asking about the reactions of significant others will serve to explore the issue of **negative entreaty** — the expression of advice on required behavioural change given in negative terms: *'Stop scratching!'* is notorious for paradoxically increasing self-damaging behaviour. Change is much better achieved by positive advice as to what *to do*, not what *not to do*. Therefore a useful slogan for parents and their children can be,

'Don't **Don't,** *Do* **Do***!'*

Covering these ideas within assessment is a useful preliminary to the introduction of behaviour modification in general, and habit reversal in particular.

Background history

The detailed protocol sets out the headings under which a full review of background history can be undertaken. Whether this is necessary or desirable will vary according to circumstances. Experience using the format given shows it can be covered quite quickly in most cases. When it becomes lengthy, issues may be highlighted that may well be relevant either to achieving successful treatment, or to understanding poor prognosis. Thus, understanding the relevance of both the parents and children of the patient also having atopic skin disease will often help the patient appreciate entrenched attitudes and behaviour patterns, and a review of personal history and personality traits may begin to show for a particular patient what may prove to be a vested interest in continuing **illness behaviour** (p. 85).

Objective findings

A preliminary objective assessment of the skin and if appropriate full physical examination, is clearly relevant to assessment — though throughout the programme itself greater emphasis is placed on **subjective** reports of skin condition, as the patient's view is emphasised. Towards the end of the first phase of the programme, when follow-up is being planned, there may be a need to confront subjective assessment with objective findings (p. 81).

Review of mental state is primarily useful for considering issues of attitude, general intelligence, rapport with the therapist, and broad behavioural characteristics best summarised as personality traits. Such observations will sometimes suggest the need for a particular approach, if good outcome is to be achieved.

Other procedures

Objective assessment of the skin condition can be supplemented usefully by photography. Furthermore biological markers, including assessment of immune status, may be useful — requiring appropriate laboratory investigations (p. 9).

Prognosis

It is always valuable as part of any clinical assessment to make a firm statement of likely prognosis. In order that vague terms are avoided, a score out of 10 can be useful — 10 being the best result possible. Thought given to the justification of prognosis is particularly helpful in formulating an appropriate management plan. If difficulties are anticipated early, they will cause less frustration later as they can then be met with strategies that are most useful for the individual patient.

4.3 The Three Levels of Treatment

The introduction of the treatment programme can usefully be made following behavioural analysis at the first visit. The first part of the patient's handbook (Appendix 2) is used to brief the patient sufficiently for a period — usually a week — of baseline registration of scratching behaviour.

Atopy and atopic skin disease

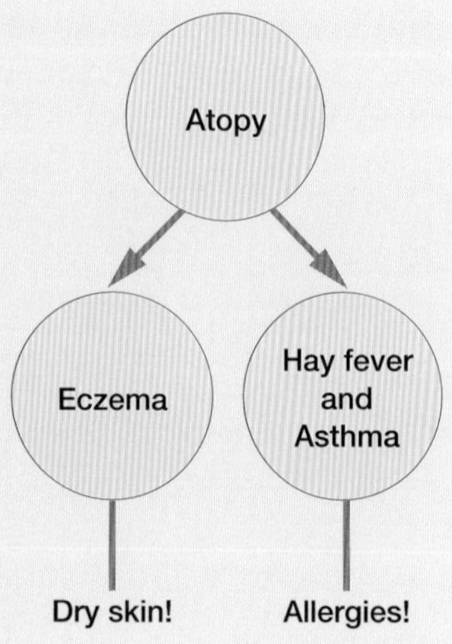

The handbook begins with a simple exposition of atopy: a constitutional predisposition to eczema, asthma and hayfever (Fig 4.8). This preliminary discussion will complement what the patient already knows, as well as giving the opportunity to correct any misconceptions. It allows also for the message to be given that 'Living with Atopy' is certainly unavoidable, but 'Living with Eczema' is certainly not.

The relevance of **dry skin** is introduced, contrasting this characteristic of atopic skin disease with the relevance of **allergy** in asthma and hay fever. The hyper-sensitivity to environmental and dietary factors experienced by patients with atopic skin disease occurs in particular when the skin is damaged — once healing has been accomplished, the skin will gradually recover its previous resistance and resilience. Allergy can unfortunately become an all-consuming preoccupation for some patients, preventing them from appreciating fully the relevance of other features of their condition, where **their own behaviour** needs to be the proper focus of their attention, and energy channelled into achieving appropriate behavioural change.

The structure of normal skin and the histology of chronic eczema

The dryness of skin in atopic skin disease leads to a consideration of the features of normal skin at microscopic level (Figs 4.9 and 4.10). A simple diagram in the patient handbook (p. 118) illustrates the regular compact nature of normal epidermal architecture. The good

Fig 4.8

Atopy

Eczema

Hay fever and Asthma

Dry skin!

Allergies!

Fig 4.9

NORMAL SKIN	CHRONIC ECZEMA
Protects against water loss	Increased porosity leads to increased water loss
Strong, yet flexible	Thickened, yet friable
Constant orderly regeneration	Chaotic cellular over-activity

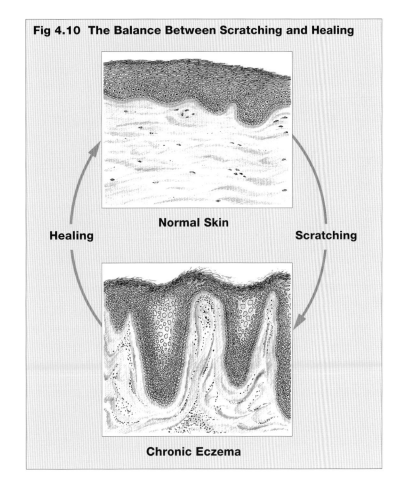

Fig 4.10 The Balance Between Scratching and Healing

Normal Skin

Healing

Scratching

Chronic Eczema

protection given by normal skin against excessive water loss, its strength-yet-flexibility and the constant process of regeneration of epidermal cells from the basal layer, are all reviewed.

In contrast the histology of skin in chronic eczema (pp. 9–10) is explained: the unevenness in thickness of the epidermis, with thin areas frequently cracking, is easily appreciated. The loss of insulation against water loss, and the chaotic appearance of the epidermal cell layers are relevant to the discussion.

The most crucial point however is to describe how non-atopic, healthy skin will take on the same characteristics of chronic eczema when experimentally damaged in the laboratory using 'a scratching machine' (p. 44). Thus the change in appearance from normal skin to that of long-standing eczema is the result of *scratching and rubbing*. However, when the scratching machine is turned off, the skin heals: within a short period normal histology reappears. Healing of skin is known to be an itchy process. As folklore has it: *'Don't scratch that itch, else you'll stop the healing'*.

This exposition of normal and abnormal histology, together with the part played by scratching and *natural healing processes*, is a central feature of the programme, and can be returned to on more than one occasion at subsequent visits to emphasise its importance.

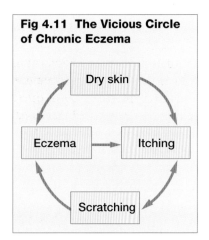

Fig 4.11 The Vicious Circle of Chronic Eczema

The vicious circle

An illustration consolidates the discussion so far, showing the close relationship between eczema and dry skin, and how both are associated with itchiness (Fig 4.11).

That itch will lead to scratch — and scratch to itch — then serves to highlight the chronic damage caused by scratching and completes a **vicious circle.** This explains why areas of skin that are easy to scratch and rub, for example the face, neck and hands are especially susceptible to chronic eczema.

Two, or three levels of treatment?

By dividing the diagram of the vicious circle, the levels of treatment required where eczema is long-standing can be introduced (Fig 4.12). Although the relevance of emollients and the role of topical steroids is usually already appreciated, such knowledge should not be taken for granted. Unfortunately even after years of use some patients fail to appreciate even the important distinction between these two treatments. They fail therefore to benefit fully from their appropriate use, as well as courting the possibility of side-effects from the inappropriate application of topical steroids.

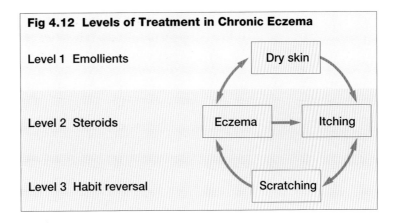

Fig 4.12 Levels of Treatment in Chronic Eczema

Level 1 Emollients

Level 2 Steroids

Level 3 Habit reversal

Dry skin — Eczema — Itching — Scratching

The levels of treatment required for the vicious circle draws attention to the fact that *'there is no cream strong enough to deal with scratching'*.

Established and habitual self-damaging behaviour can maintain the chronicity of atopic skin disease, regardless of any topical or systemic treatment. In contrast, when atopic eczema has newly appeared and is dealt with promptly, appropriate and thorough treatment with moisturisers and topical steroids can be totally effective. The contrast between old, established chronic atopic skin disease with new, recently appeared eczema allows for further review of the aim of the treatment programme. Proper management including at Level 3, **habit reversal**, frees the patient from chronicity, with subsequent relapses being managed using only conventional treatment at Levels 1 and 2 — **emollients** and **topical steroids** — in such a way that further chronicity is avoided.

Scratching and registration

The discussion of scratching behaviour in the assessment process is now taken further. All touching, rubbing and picking of the skin is to count — and be counted — as scratching. It has already been pointed out that although itching provokes scratching, scratching not only becomes a relatively unconscious behaviour over time, it also becomes associated with particular situations, circumstances and activities. Even without itch, such environmental factors will predictably provoke self-damaging behaviour. Sometimes it is only after scratching has begun that itching complicates the situation.

In order to address a long-standing habit it is necessary as a first step to create a conscious awareness of the

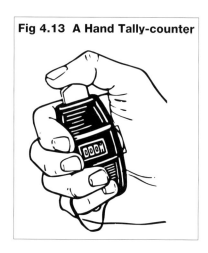

Fig 4.13 A Hand Tally-counter

behaviour in question. Baseline registration of the frequency of the habit is therefore the important next step. The introduction of the hand tally-counter (Fig 4.13) usually provokes a smile with raised eyebrows, and serves to underline the necessary interest that is to be taken in what is actually happening between the patient and their skin in everyday life away from the consulting room.

That counting scratching frequencies will take trouble, and will interfere with the flow of things at home, and at work, will be offset by pointing out that it introduces a small but necessary element of self-discipline. It is helpful to clarify that habit reversal is only required to deal with the chronic syndrome: after a few weeks it will become unnecessary.

It is useful to demonstrate the use of the tally-counter. Each 'batch' of scratching should be counted, rather than each scratch 'stroke'. The hand goes to the skin, scratches, comes away again and presses the counter once for one 'scratching', rather than several times for several 'scratches'. A simultaneous two-handed scratch therefore counts two, for 'two scratchings'. **All touching, rubbing and picking** need registration. The tally-counter should be carried at all times, and used immediately — it is not as effective to 'remember' a few scratches and add them to the tally-counter later. The patient is asked to bring the tally-counter to subsequent visits. During an interview any scratching should be counted. This behaviour is noted and therefore reinforced by the interviewer.

At the end of 24 hours the total on the tally-counter is to be recorded in the handbook, and the counter then reset to zero. The best time for this can be in the evening, before bed. During initial registration it is important to advise that **scratching is not to be avoided** — registration introduces self discipline as well as increasing awareness of scratching behaviour. Once the treatment programme has started **continuing registration** of scratching not only maintains awareness but also monitors progress.

During registration the provocative situations, circumstances and activities associated with scratching become increasingly obvious (Fig 4.14). These should be noted for further discussion. Scratching during sleep is a common phenomenon. It leaves blood on the bed linen, wakes the patient, and disturbs others. It is not expected that the frequency of scratching during sleep can be registered. Responsibility for scratching is only to be taken

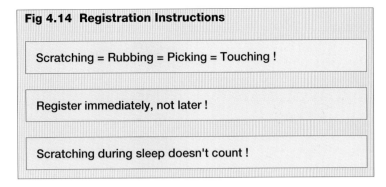

Fig 4.14 Registration Instructions

> Scratching = Rubbing = Picking = Touching !

> Register immediately, not later !

> Scratching during sleep doesn't count !

during the day and the evening — not when asleep. If the situations during wakefulness are dealt with effectively healing will begin and night-time scratching will resolve without any other intervention. For the occasional patient who asserts that they only scratch at night, it is important to persist with the registration exercise. It will, with the help of others at home and at work, demonstrate to them that it is awareness of scratching, and not scratching itself that has been absent during the day.

During the registration period, the conventional treatment to date can be continued. It is reviewed and revised when habit reversal instruction is given at the next visit. As well as asking the patient to bring their tally-counter to the next visit, they should bring with them also their handbook, as it will be frequently referred and added to.

Review of registration and patients observations

It is natural to begin the second consultation by considering the 'homework' that has been carried out. Enthusiasm for this assignment varies, and may reflect the chances of a good outcome. Otherwise, paying close attention to what has been achieved will reinforce the patient's efforts so far.

The relationship of scratching frequency to subjective (and objective) disease severity is by no means straightforward. However, the impression is gained that the higher the reported scratching frequencies, the more likely the patient will do well with the programme — reflecting their commitment and enthusiasm for what has been already covered. Some with high frequencies do not do well however, while some with low results achieve a great deal.

The first week's daily registrations can be copied out for future reference. Figures that are 'rounded up' are clearly less 'authentic' than those showing a natural variability. The additionally reported particular antecedents of scratching are noted for further discussion.

Review of behaviour and skin status

At this and each subsequent visit, a series of direct questions can help set the scene for discussion. In addition to recording the registration of frequencies (at subsequent visits this can be limited to the last 7 days) and the most **scratchy situations**, the percentage of scratching that comes from itch is reviewed again. With increasing awareness of habitual behaviour, the reported percentage of scratching **not** provoked by itch may well have increased. It is important to allow discussion of this and other new observations arising from the homework.

Three questions concerning behaviour are matched by three questions on subjective skin status — the patient's severity score using a 0–10 range as in initial assessment, the noting of where the skin is affected, and finally a discussion of how much of the eczema is long-standing as opposed to relatively new (Fig 4.15).

The three levels of treatment

Part 2 of the handbook begins with a reminder of the vicious circle diagram divided into three levels of treatment (p. 61). It is most important to emphasise that the approach attaches prime significance to using both habit reversal techniques **and usual somatic treatments**. Not only are these all combined, but each level is considered from the behavioural point of view — effective somatic treatment depends on appropriate patient behaviour as much as the innovation of habit reversal.

A preliminary summary of the main features of each level of treatment is therefore valuable in explaining the need to consider the use of emollients, and topical steroids in some detail, before introducing the habit reversal itself.

Level 1: emollient therapy

The proper use of moisturisers should be based on an understanding of what is involved. The structure of healthy, and damaged skin has already been introduced. A diagram in the patient handbook helps to illustrate the continuous

---

Fig 4.15 Progress Review

- Frequency of scratching

- Scratching situations

- % Scratching from itch

- Subjective score 0–10

- Parts affected

- % Long-standing vs. recent

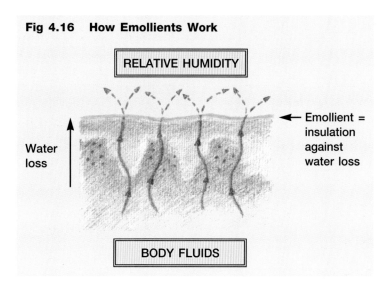

Fig 4.16 How Emollients Work

RELATIVE HUMIDITY

Water loss

Emollient = insulation against water loss

BODY FLUIDS

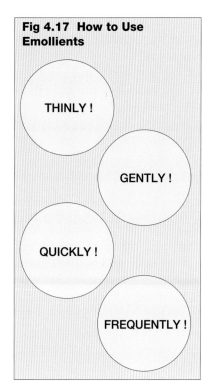

Fig 4.17 How to Use Emollients

THINLY !

GENTLY !

QUICKLY !

FREQUENTLY !

passage of water from deeper tissues, through the skin and into the surrounding air and how body temperature, and relative humidity of the air, as well as skin condition will influence the need for emollients (Fig 4.16).

The surface 'pavement cells' are 'cemented together' — and in eczema 'the cement' is deficient, and allows water to 'leak out' of the skin at a greater than usual rate, causing the skin to dry. The need is for a **thin** layer of grease on the skin, **gently** and **quickly** applied without fuss. A thick layer ('like a cross-channel swimmer') serves also to keep heat in and cause discomfort, while emollient applied with rubbing offers potential trauma to fragile skin — a gentle wipe on of the smallest amount is sufficient — *'a shine is all that's needed'* (Fig 4.17).

If the use of emollients is referred to as 'prevention' rather than 'treatment', the need to apply them **frequently** and proactively can be better appreciated. The question *'when do you use emollients?'*, will usually elicit the obvious response *'when my skin is dry!'*. For prophylaxis, this is clearly **too late**. Pacing the application of moisturiser is therefore a behaviour of relevance in optimising treatment, as is the use of the full range of emollient therapy. In order to establish the preferred applications a trial pack can be used (p. 155).

Exposed areas such as the face, neck and hands may need very frequent emollient treatment at the beginning of the programme, i.e. hourly. Such treatment, applied gently, itself provides a practical alternative to scratching (see Level 3, p. 67).

As well as clarifying for a few patients the distinction between emollient and topical steroid treatments, the way they are used separately or together needs review. Emollients are to be used as frequently as necessary to keep the skin moist — the frequency will vary according to the area of body, severity of condition and the use of steroids. Emollients will be used **on their own**, and **with topical steroids** — but topical steroids are not to be used on their own.

When used together the topical steroid is to be applied first, with the emollient applied second, as a dressing (pp. 22–23).

Level 2: topical steroids

There are two particular aspects of topical steroid treatment to address with all patients, and both are associated with the common wariness that exists towards potential side-effects. They are (a) using **too weak** a steroid, and (b) **stopping too soon**.

The strength of the steroid used needs to be appropriate to the task required — a definite and complete healing effect is needed. Once the skin has thoroughly healed, the topical steroid is discontinued. Reviewing the use of steroid treatment to date will often reveal use of steroids at inadequate strengths. Coupled with self-damaging behaviour such sub-optimal treatment leads to development of the chronic syndrome. Using a steroid at an adequate strength — with moisturiser and habit reversal — will bring the best results. There will be then less overall use of steroids in the long term, reducing rather than increasing the risk of side-effects.

A simple diagram is used in order to understand how long to apply the steroid (Fig 4.18). This shows 'the healing curve'. When the curve hits the base-line, the skin 'looks good'. It is then that most patients immediately discontinue treatment with topical steroids. However, with topical treatment the skin heals in two stages, from outside in. At the 'Look Good Point' the eczema might seem to have cleared, but it is actually still present under the surface as an inflammatory infiltrate in the dermis. When topical steroids are stopped at this point a relapse soon follows: the eczema can be described as 'bubbling up and over' again. Up to the 'Look Good Point' healing has been 'obvious' (or **cosmetic**). A further period of topical steroid treatment

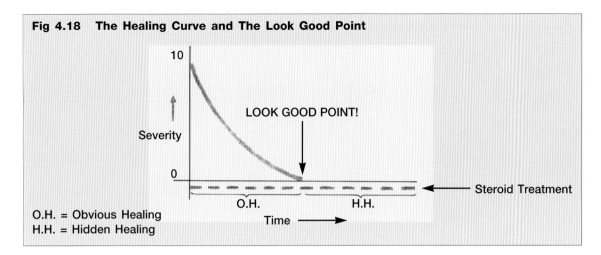

Fig 4.18   The Healing Curve and The Look Good Point

Severity — 10 ... LOOK GOOD POINT! ... 0

O.H.   H.H.

Time

Steroid Treatment

O.H. = Obvious Healing
H.H. = Hidden Healing

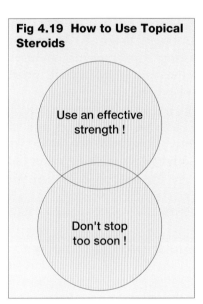

Fig 4.19 How to Use Topical Steroids

Use an effective strength !

Don't stop too soon !

on the same skin is needed to accomplish 'hidden' (or **histological**) healing — how long this period of treatment will be needed might need a trial-and-error approach, but a rule of thumb is to say it is as long as it took to get to the 'Look Good Point', using all three levels of treatment appropriately. This may be another two or three weeks in some cases, though the frequency and strength of topical steroid for histological healing may be reduced latterly (Fig 4.19).

In our protocol the patient usually returns for review in two weeks time for their third visit, so it is sufficient to advise that the newly prescribed steroid treatment should be continued until then, even if the skin 'looks good' in the meantime.

Level 3: habit reversal

Principles of behaviour modification
As with Levels 1 and 2, the handbook helps explain Level 3, **habit reversal**. It is useful to spend time initially discussing the principles of **behaviour modification** in the simplest terms. Thus, as an essential first step, there needs to be a behaviour, clearly defined, that it is agreed needs changing. Hopefully the programme so far has established this. Registration will have made the patient more aware of the behaviour, and the base-line frequency will have been established, together with its most common antecedents.

Using the A, B, and C of Antecedents, Behaviour and Consequences, the sequential way of 'understanding' the behaviour is introduced (Fig 4.20).

67

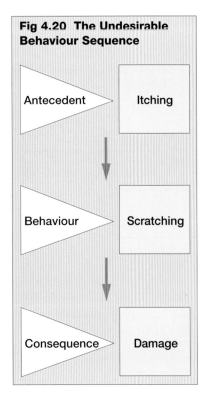

Fig 4.20 The Undesirable Behaviour Sequence

The established sequence needs interruption to allow a different **consequence**; with no further damage, **healing** occurs. Thus new **behaviour** is needed after the **antecedent** (**itch**), such that when it is performed the **behaviour** : Scratch is no longer possible. Hence the new **consequence** (**healing**) will be achieved (Fig 4.21).

Specific instructions

Scratching is divided into two behavioural stages: (a) 'going to' the area to be scratched, and (b) scratching. This is described in the handbook, and should be demonstrated to the patient. Scratching is **old**, undesirable behaviour, to be replaced be **new**, desirable behaviour — desirable because the consequence will be healing.

Stage (a) of the new behaviour is **clenching the fists gently for 30 seconds**, fixing the arms in a comfortable position at the sides of the body. Stage (b) is **gentle pinching or pressing of a finger nail** against the area of skin that would otherwise have been scratched, **until the impulse to scratch has gone**.

The new behaviour should be demonstrated, doing it together with the patient. The handbook sets out a sequence for the patient to practice (p. 127), a few times over the next two days. Otherwise from now on all scratching is to be replaced by the new sequence. If the relevant antecedents to scratching are referred to as **impulses**, the point that it is not only itching that provokes scratching is emphasised again. The patient is advised that if the **impulse to scratch** goes during the 30 seconds of fist clenching, there is no need to go on to the new stage (b), skin pinching or pressing with a finger nail.

In designing this particular new behavioural sequence 'habit-scratching' is seen as being countered by fist clenching, and the 'itch-scratching' is seen as being replaced by skin pinching or finger nail pressing. If this is explained, some patients will remember learning as children how the itch of an insect bite can be relieved by briefly pressing a finger nail into the wheal caused by the bite (p. 45).

General strategies

The handbook goes on to explain how to alter behaviour more generally — how to limit, and eliminate damage caused by scratching using more general measures. Thus when the circumstances during which scratching seems

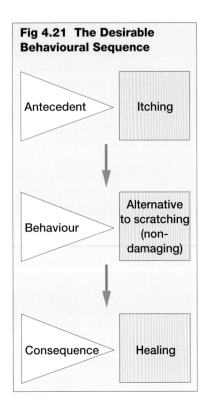

Fig 4.21 The Desirable Behavioural Sequence

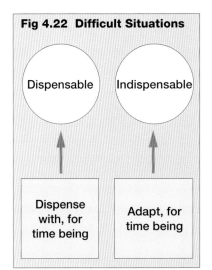

Fig 4.22 Difficult Situations

Dispensable | Indispensable

Dispense with, for time being | Adapt, for time being

to occur are reviewed, a first step is to agree which of these are indispensable, and which for the time being (two to four weeks) can be dispensed with, or avoided (Fig 4.22). Those situations and activities that are unavoidable, and associated with scratching, will invariably have characteristics that can be modified, to reduce the chance of self-damage. The handbook gives several examples of such modifications (p. 128). These usually involve one or more of three main tactics (Fig 4.23) (Plates 4.2 and 4.3).

Using this advice, the patient is asked to (a) decide on how they are going to divide up their difficult situations into the indispensable and dispensable categories, and (b) to write out a list of tactics in their handbook, for dealing with those circumstances or activities that are evidently indispensable. This list of desirable behaviours can then be referred to as their **behavioural prescription**, and it should be reviewed regularly at subsequent visits.

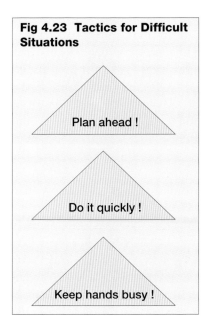

Fig 4.23 Tactics for Difficult Situations

Plan ahead !

Do it quickly !

Keep hands busy !

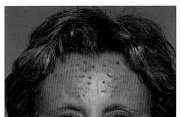

Plate 4.2 Healing through habit reversal — an atopic patient's forehead before. . .

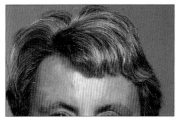

Plate 4.3 . . . and after adopting knitting 'to keep hands busy while watching television' — an effective patient modifiation of the habit reversal technique.

These tactics are particularly useful for those situations in which carrying out the specific habit reversal instructions would not be practical.

Instructions

Using the patient handbook, written instructions can be given for all three levels of the programme. The use of topical steroids during the first two weeks after registration is charted by the patient, to increase compliance. Experience suggests that it is definitely worthwhile

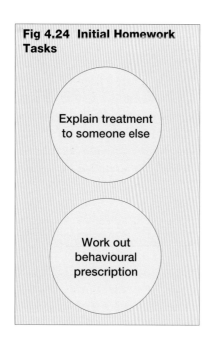

Fig 4.24 Initial Homework Tasks

Explain treatment to someone else

Work out behavioural prescription

providing clear written instructions on what to use and when to use it; the instructions are recorded separately in the case file for future reference. At Level 3, registration of any further scratching is continued over the next four weeks at least, to note progress. It is necessary to explain carefully that registration is only required for **scratching** and not for the new alternative and desirable behaviours.

The **behavioural prescription** is worked out by the patient after the second visit. It is useful to suggest also that the patient should now describe the programme in detail to another person away from the clinic (Fig 4.24). If they find explaining what is involved difficult, they should note down what has become unclear, and bring back their notes to the next visit for discussion.

4.4 Three Further Dimensions in Management

Stress

Asking about stress sometimes feels like risking the opening of Pandora's box. The topic is often avoided as it may pose problems for the interviewer who feels therapeutically impotent. In reality a sympathetic appraisal of this topic for each patient need not pose problems, and can often be very useful. During initial assessment there can be review of factors that either improve or provoke eczema.

Not all patients report stress as relevant. Of those that do, some report that it is **during stress**, for example examinations, that the effect is most noticeable — others interestingly assert it is in the period **after stress** has passed that their eczema seems to relapse. Either way, discussing how to manage stress is relevant. Stress and eczema are clearly linked in a **reciprocal relationship**, and this phenomenon is common to the relationship between morbid emotional states and all three of the common dermatoses — eczema, psoriasis and acne. A first principle should be to manage the skin condition appropriately and effectively, taking into account the particular needs of the individual patient. This in itself relieves stress, and improves morale: the patient who is managing their skin well will be better able to manage their life, and the inevitable stressful events that all lives involve.

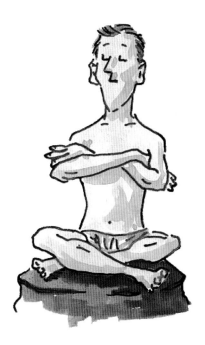

First aid for coping with stress can be provided by any health professional, and the use of written material is most useful here. A list of tactics (p. 158) which can be helpful is worth reviewing with some patients, adding the suggestion that the list be discussed with others at home. Particularly useful ideas for the individual can be discussed further at a future visit. The tactics listed can be reduced to **three Golden Rules**: regular opportunities for favourite relaxing activities, consideration of the various spheres of the individual's life to ensure there is a sensible balance, and lastly enquiring if coping with stress involves counter-productive habits, for example excessive coffee intake, or over-use of alcohol (Fig 4.25).

Anxiety management training will be worth considering for a small number of patients who have ingrained inappropriate responses to stress, that fail to respond to the simpler interventions above, and evidently require extra help. Such **behavioural psychotherapy** requires the involvement of appropriately trained professional help, as does the occasional need for **psychodynamic psychotherapy**. When the latter is indicated, it may be via either group or individual therapy: a preliminary psychological or psychiatric assessment is then evidently relevant.

Attitudes — of the patient

Throughout the programme importance is attached to the recognition of counter-productive attitudes held by the patient. Assessment of attitude is in part achieved by direct discussion, and also by incidental observation of chance remarks. However, we can generally safely assume that most patients will have been conditioned by previous experience to become fatalistic about their eczema, and to regard conventional treatments as palliative, if not relatively useless, and in the case of steroids, offering more risk of side-effects than any worthwhile good effects. As a result of these entrenched beliefs, the patient's attempts to cope with eczema can seem poorly coordinated, and even illogical in execution. There is an often held view that eczema needs to be **accepted and lived with** — especially when its 'not too bad'. While these views can be evident from the start, and should be gently confronted throughout the programme, they can be especially relevant later when, despite appropriate instruction, recalcitrant areas of long-standing eczema remain.

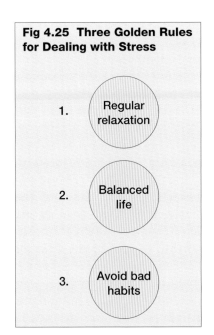

Fig 4.25 Three Golden Rules for Dealing with Stress

1. Regular relaxation

2. Balanced life

3. Avoid bad habits

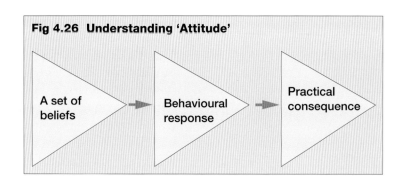

Fig 4.26 Understanding 'Attitude'

A set of beliefs → Behavioural response → Practical consequence

---

Fig 4.27 Key Messages

Confront beliefs!

•

Suggest new behaviour!

•

Focus on desirable consequences

There are three possible processes for achieving **attitudinal change**, reflecting the essential qualities of 'attitude'. An attitude can be best understood as a belief or set of beliefs that dictates particular overt behaviour, which in itself has certain more or less predictable consequences (Fig 4.26).

Using these three components in turn we can (a) confront beliefs directly, (b) give advice on appropriate behavioural change, and lastly (c) focus on desirable consequences that occur with such change, reinforcing then appropriate behaviour and positive attitudes (Fig 4.27).

Thus active participation in the programme is to be encouraged for all patients, from the beginning. There is a need to stress the importance of what happens between the patient and their skin when they are **not** in the clinic — when they are at home, at school or at work. They are now encouraged to regard their own behaviour, based on a fresh understanding of their condition and its management, as of the greatest relevance. One direct attitudinal intervention is to offer the advice, *'Manage, don't be managed'*.

Frequent opportunities arise throughout the programme to emphasise that success depends on the patient's own efforts — at all levels of treatment — both during spoken transactions, and in the written material taken away.

As the programme progresses both the interactional style of the approach, and the need now to carry out particular new behaviours based on explained rationale, involving all levels of treatment, is central to changing attitude. Then as attitude begins to change — what is said, and what is achieved will be the indicators — the new ideas need nurturing, encouraging and reinforcing. As the condition responds to the programme, progress is overtly measured, with the improvement clearly linked to the patient's new ways of coping. It becomes evident that **taking the trouble is worth the effort**.

Habits are not only seen in overt behaviour: habit reversal is needed also in the ways of understanding and thinking about atopic skin disease — both by the patient, and by others.

Attitudes — of others

Although feelings of impotence and pessimism come partly from the frustrating experience of long-term disability itself, the testimony of people with eczema points also to the relevance of attitudes of other people. These external influences include cultural factors generally, and views evidently originating in family life, especially during childhood. However, when some recollections of experiences of consulting professionals, including specialists, are considered, an important source of unnecessary difficulty becomes evident. Clearly the impotence felt by an advisor can be quickly transferred unwittingly to the person being advised; helplessness is contagious, and any useful advice that is offered will then end up quickly being forgotten as the patient leaves the consultation demoralised and depressed about their condition.

In tackling this unhappy phenomenon with our patients, we take a first step by acknowledging that it is regrettably a real and relevant factor, and then go on to discuss how it needs careful handling. We explain how it is both possible and necessary to achieve a certain immunity to such negative influences, through both a greater personal understanding of what is required and also of how to get the best out of the professional help available. Each patient with atopic skin disease benefits from learning as much as possible about their condition, including the evident controversies that inevitably exist. Thus the patient can become his or her **own expert**, whilst working with the professional help available in a collaborative way. It is then possible to achieve the best possible results in the management of their own condition.

For the professionals themselves there are two important issues. First, there needs to be a good understanding of the causes of long-standing atopic skin disease, and through that an understanding of a more rational and effective approach to management. Secondly, we recommend a return to the treatment of each patient **as a whole person**, with appropriate attention to the relevance of constructive support and encouragement, if the more potent treatments that are now available are to be made as effective as possible. It is ironic that otherwise the alienation that seems so characteristic of being a patient in the latter part of the 20th century leads to neglect of the good treatments available, and the search for solace with alternative therapies offered by herbalists and other non-scientific traditional healers from other cultures.

4.5 Follow-up

Early

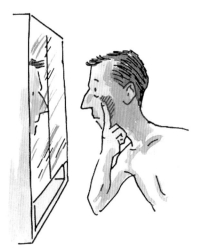

Following our protocol, the treatment instructions are completed by the end of the second consultation. The early follow-up at the third appointment, together with the fourth visit, monitors progress in treatment at all the three levels detailed above. Each time the patient attends they should bring with them their handbook and record of progress. Registration of scratching should show a frequency of less than 20 per day by the fourth visit.

Review

At each of these visits it is helpful first to focus on a review of scratching behaviour noting scratching frequency over the last seven days, the situations when it is most troublesome, and from the patient's point of view how much of the scratching is still coming from itch. Then the focus turns to the eczema itself, noting the severity again from the patient's point of view on the scale 0–10 as before, where the rash is to be found, and finally the proportion of the eczema that is old and long-standing, as opposed to newly arrived (p. 53). If these six points are recorded at each visit, the record becomes standardised and can be more easily reviewed subsequently (p. 64, Fig 4.15).

Treatment review

Progress in treatment can then be discussed by taking each level of treatment in turn. At each level there is a need to review the rationale, and ensure that the best possible results are being achieved. It is helpful to check how much is understood by direct questions. Reviewing the basics is essential, as they are rarely absorbed thoroughly first time round.

Review of difficult situations, and habit reversal

As the scratching frequency falls, often the proportion due to itch increases. However, situations and circumstances remain strikingly relevant and the use of a diagram of two 12 hour clock faces, one for the day and another for the night, makes it possible to document the hours and situations when most damage is still being done (Fig 4.28).

When scratching is less than 50 episodes per day the difficult times usually become particularly localised, e.g. first thing in the morning, early evening and last thing at night. Showing that this is the case gives an opportunity for encouraging the patient, concentrating their efforts to practise the new appropriate behaviours at particular times, therefore limiting and finally eliminating self-damaging behaviour. This will seem a feasible proposition, as it involves perhaps only three or four hours out of the total 24 each day. The time commitment involved in habit reversal needs to be kept in perspective for the patient; compared with the endless treatment procedures experienced to date, habit reversal is a time limited intervention. It will be effective in two to four weeks, and should never be required again if subsequently follow-up advice is adhered to successfully.

The difficult times will draw attention again to the patient's own **behavioural prescription**; discussion will encourage the patient, and their own particular

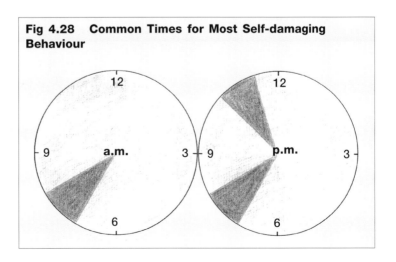

Fig 4.28   Common Times for Most Self-damaging Behaviour

techniques might be worth noting for future reference when advising others. Looking at circumstances is the main opportunity for considering the general advice that has been given, but the specific habit reversal technique should also be reviewed. Most find it satisfactory as it is, while others will develop their own preferred variations. Here the guiding rule should be **'whatever works'** — certainly innovative tactics can be reinforced, as they indicate the patients motivation to take control and manage their own condition. By taking responsibility they increase the likelihood of getting the best results.

The healing curve

A graphic demonstration of how progress is achieved helps to emphasise that though nothing can be achieved without habit reversal, the appropriate application of treatment at Levels 1 and 2 are also essential for complete healing, and all three levels involve the patient's own active effort (Fig 4.29).

Trouble shooting

At follow-up a variety of issues may need consideration. Sometimes these problems are obvious, but sometimes they only become apparent through direct questioning.

The relevance of **stress** may have been identified at assessment. As the skin heals, the need for particular advice will become evident, and how much help is appropriate will need to be decided. **Forgotten areas**

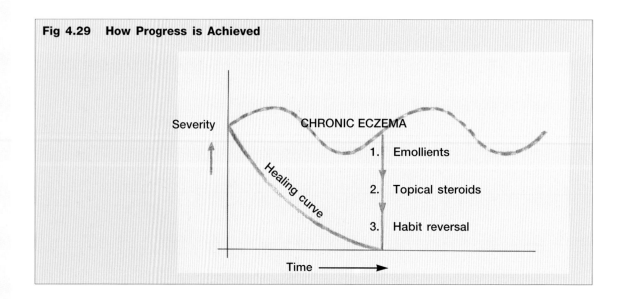

Fig 4.29   How Progress is Achieved

are worth considering regularly and will need to be specifically asked about — some patches of chronic eczema seem to become 'old friends' and there can be a tenacious desire to hold on to them. The rationale for clearing the skin completely can be considered, as detailed below (p. 80).

Infections and **sensitivities** (pp. 37–42) can interrupt smooth progress in treatment. When they do they provide an opportunity for the patient to learn more about management, and this will be helpful for the future. Because it has happened before does not necessarily mean that the patient fully understands the problem. What might seem obvious still needs explanation. Understanding the relevance of finding appropriate user-friendly topical treatments, and how to recognise and effectively treat infection keeps the patient's attitude positive and proactive.

Healing, and continuing registration

The fourth visit of our protocol sees the patient about four weeks after full treatment has begun — and by now some report the skin has healed, though for most another one or two weeks may be required. Usually registration of scratching frequency can be maintained up to the fourth visit, and some are happy to continue further. At the fourth visit further registration can either be abandoned, or can be used now in a random way. If discontinued, it can be introduced later if a 'refresher' element seems indicated.

Hidden healing

As the skin heals the instruction on topical steroid treatment needs careful review. Achieving 'hidden' healing (p. 26) is important, but finally discontinuing the use of topical steroids also needs emphasis, especially as a stronger preparation may have been introduced for this programme.

Scratching frequencies, and focus of habit reversal

By the fourth visit habit reversal will have reduced scratching frequencies often to less than 10 episodes per day: that should certainly be the aim. For most patients this means almost all the scratching is now provoked by itch. The success of a focus for habit reversal, as introduced at the third visit, should be reviewed during the

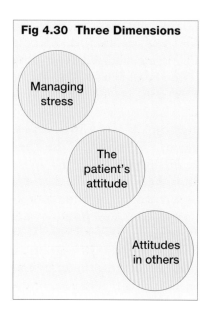

Fig 4.30 Three Dimensions

Managing stress

The patient's attitude

Attitudes in others

fourth visit to reinforce the importance of eliminating all self-damaging behaviour.

The three dimensions

Before arranging longer term follow-up, the 'three dimensions' should be considered (Fig 4.30). How much time is spent on this will vary considerably. The majority of patients report that the programme gives them significant 'mastery' over their condition and as a result they feel more confident in coping with stress, and are evidently more generally optimistic and positive in their attitude. It is however useful to recommend again a **proactive** approach to stress management, if stress has been an important cause of relapse in the past. It is relevant also for all 'graduates' of the programme to understand how to cope positively in the future when meeting negative attitudes in others. We help by keeping in close touch with the relevant primary health care team, ensuring as far as possible that they are well informed of the principles of our programme — especially for follow-up (p. 159).

Discontinuing levels of treatment

Using a version of the 'healing curve' diagram it can be shown how the levels of treatment in the combined approach are sequentially discontinued: habit reversal becomes unnecessary first, soon after the 'Look Good Point'. Level 2 treatment continues until 'hidden' healing is judged complete. Level 1 treatment continues longer, though not necessarily indefinitely (Fig 4.31). With recovery, the skin can regain its normal water–retaining characteristics.

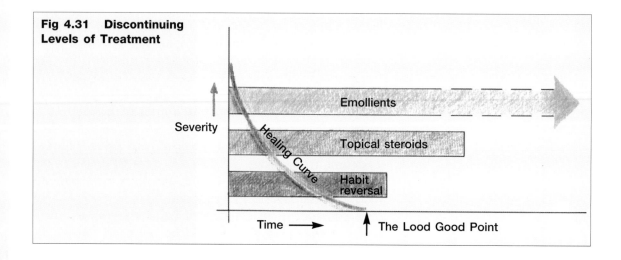

Fig 4.31 Discontinuing Levels of Treatment

Severity

Emollients

Healing Curve

Topical steroids

Habit reversal

Time ⟶   The Lood Good Point

Fig 4.32 Relapse Recognition

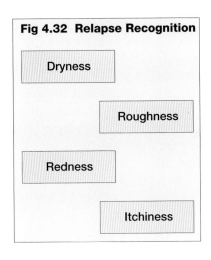

Dryness

Roughness

Redness

Itchiness

Relapse recognition

In place of continuous topical treatment there needs now to be **continuous vigilance** for signs of relapse. These are listed in the handbook. It needs emphasising there should be a low tolerance of relapse: if a relapse is suspected it should be treated vigorously. Dryness and roughness indicate need for emollient therapy; redness and itching indicate the need for treatment with steroids and emollients (Fig 4.32).

The causes of relapse should be reviewed. It is worth discussing how some factors behind eczema are 'continuous' and ever present, e.g. atopy itself, while others are relatively 'intermittent', for example season or climate, or stress. Thus a relapse will occur when, in addition to the continuous influences there are a number of intermittent factors at any one time — but once this has been effectively treated the intermittent factors may no longer be operating. Treatment can then be discontinued without a further relapse occurring.

Treating relapses

Reference to the vicious circle (p. 60) of long-standing atopic skin disease helps explain that when dealing with an acute relapse uncomplicated by scratching, only vigorous treatment at Levels 1 and 2 is necessary. A good response can be expected in a relatively short period of time. We give our patients an 'off the shelf' standard approach for dealing with relapses, together with the advice that it can be adapted for individual requirements (Fig 4.33).

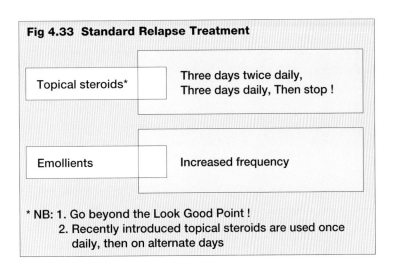

Fig 4.33 Standard Relapse Treatment

| Topical steroids* | Three days twice daily, Three days daily, Then stop ! |
| Emollients | Increased frequency |

* NB: 1. Go beyond the Look Good Point !
2. Recently introduced topical steroids are used once daily, then on alternate days

Assuming that when the relapse occurs a topical steroid is not being used, the application of an effective topical steroid twice a day for three days and then once a day for three days together with an increased frequency of use of moisturiser should produce good healing within the treatment period — the **Look Good Point** will occur within the first two or three days. As with healing in long-term atopic skin disease, for the relapse there are two stages for healing — obvious, and hidden. It is important when giving instructions on treating relapses to review the principles behind emollient and topical steroid treatment.

Convalescent phase

During the three months or so following effective treatment of long-standing atopic skin disease, the skin is best described as 'settling down'. As time progresses there should be less chance of relapse, with each relapse becoming less troublesome and more easy to treat. The skin becomes more tolerant of external insult, developing greater resistance and resilience. This third phase of healing may be called **invisible**, or **humoral** (p. 98, Fig 5.13).

Need for complete healing

Perhaps more important than any other factor at the follow-up stage is the importance of reviewing how **complete healing is the aim of treatment.** Old attitudes die hard and **living with a little bit** of eczema is a very tempting prospect for many patients, rather than clearing the skin completely. Three main arguments can be useful in persuading the patient to aim for perfection (Fig 4.34).

First, continuing eczema will, even for a small area, mean continuing use of topical treatments and if this involves topical steroids, the risk of side-effects. It is only by clearing the skin completely that treatment can definitely become a discontinuous and intermittent procedure. Secondly, if patches of eczema remain, the affected skin remains unstable, sensitive and more liable to relapse. The convalescent period is therefore never passed through, and the benefits that follow it never achieved. Thirdly, achieving a completely clear skin free from long-standing atopic dermatitis, perhaps for the first time in a long time, should be associated with a profound 'feel-good factor'. The patient is no longer a victim, but is much more in control and managing their condition. They can *live without eczema.*

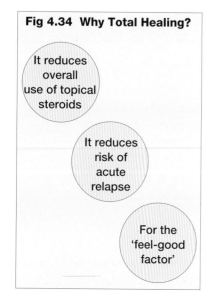

Fig 4.34 Why Total Healing?

It reduces overall use of topical steroids

It reduces risk of acute relapse

For the 'feel-good factor'

Later

Arrangements for future review

The energetic and interactive work of this combined conventional and behavioural approach emphasises investment of time and trouble, both by the patient and therapist, during the first five or six weeks of our programme. The goal of treatment comes later, and insofar as it is **healed skin** and the **elimination of chronic illness**, with the patient enjoying the fruits of their labours, later follow-up visits can be an important opportunity to review this new lease of life. Some patients will disappear from view, but others are glad to keep in touch, and benefit from doing so. Appointments can be arranged at three and six months, and then at yearly intervals.

Habit reversal at later follow-up

The skin should now be prone only to new and therefore relatively acute eczema. Management does not require registration of scratching frequency, or any analysis of self-damaging behaviours; habit reversal tactics are no longer required. Should there be a slip back into chronicity — anything lasting longer than a couple of weeks might count — a 'refresher course' of a few days registration, followed by a week or so of habit reversal, together with topical emollients and steroids, brings the condition under good control again.

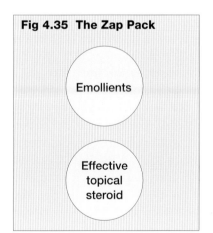

Fig 4.35 The Zap Pack

Emollients

Effective topical steroid

Need for further treatment

Treatment of relapses during this later follow-up period is, as explained above, at Levels 1 and 2 only — emollients and topical steroids. Level 2 is intermittent, and Level 1 either continuous or intermittent, depending on individual needs. In order that the response to relapse can be prompt, the patient should have available at home a **Zap Pack** of appropriate emollient and topical steroids (Fig 4.35).

The strength of the topical steroid used in the treatment of this acute eczema can be stronger than was used previously in the management of the chronic state before the patient started the combined approach programme, as its use will be time-limited.

Vigilance

From now on what is needed is **vigilance**, and a **proactive approach**. By understanding what factors are likely to provoke a relapse, some patients can alter relevant arrangements in a preventative way, reducing the risks involved (p. 99). Hence, during the winter, when relapse is more common, prophylactic principles of stress management can have greater relevance and may stop trouble before it occurs, or reduce the severity of a relapse. Confidence in self-diagnosis — using the simple symptom and sign inventory (p. 79) is clearly important, together with the confident use of the acute treatment regime.

Quality of life

Perhaps the greatest reinforcer of the newly acquired behaviours relevant to successful convalescence and future positive outcome is the improvement in **quality of life**. Our cohort reports improvements in all domains, from the most private and personal to the most public and social (Fig 4.36).

Improvements in mood and sleep are common early experiences, together with increase in self-confidence and general well-being. A greater repertoire of clothes will be worn — women may abandon trousers in favour of skirts and dresses — and general social restrictions imposed by self-consciousness are replaced by an extending repertoire of activities, including a broader variety of leisure and sporting pursuits. Swimming can be one of the first welcome new activities to become possible. With improved self-confidence, relationships with others clearly benefit. At the most intimate level, sexuality becomes an easier arena. Pain and discomfort, as well as embarrassment over appearance, are no longer significant handicaps. Family life becomes significantly more relaxed — others at home who have worried for and cared for the sufferer are relieved of their concerns. In general terms the normalisation of the home environment is a profound and welcome relief for everyone. Outside the home, at school, college, and at work there is more time, energy and self-confidence to get on with life. Courses that had been put off or not considered are now taken on, jobs that seemed out of the question are applied for and promotion and increased responsibility now seem easy to take in one's stride.

All these social repercussions may seem beyond the usual focus of therapeutic concern, but this success is secondary to achieving the attitudinal and behavioural changes that are the primary targets of The Combined Approach. Attention to these important benefits

---

Fig 4.36 Quality of Life Effects

Mood, sleep

Clothing

Activities

Relationships

Family life

Education

Employment

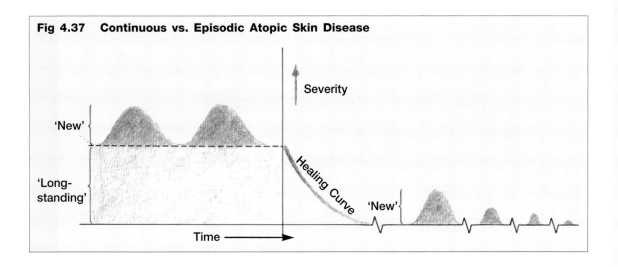

Fig 4.37   Continuous vs. Episodic Atopic Skin Disease

encourages and maintains the significant new ways of coping the patient has recently learnt.

The difference between **living with eczema** and **living without eczema** is now clearer than at any other time — passive acceptance of a chronic disability is replaced by an active and thorough tackling of the condition, such that months and perhaps years of misery are now replaced by only days of inconvenience (Fig 4.37). While eczema will still be an occasional problem, considerable stretches of life are now eczema-free: living **without** eczema is a reality.

4.6 Difficult Cases

The Combined Approach to atopic skin disease is profoundly rewarding for patients and therapists, but this does not mean everyone benefits completely from the programme. For about 20% of patients seen so far the programme proves unsuccessful, with another 20% evidently benefitting less than might be reasonably expected. Moreover, our results are influenced by the manner in which patients have been referred to us: the more clearly our programme is understood by a referrer, the more likely it is that the referral is appropriate and the outcome successful.

For some patients there is a 'biological' difficulty in benefitting from the programme. Such patients seem to be particularly sensitive to allergens in the environment, including their food. Even with such difficulties everyone with long-term and chronic atopic eczema can benefit from our approach. It is important therefore to summarise what we now think we know about those that do less well than others. Apart from the general influences already referred to, such as reluctance to use topical steroids adequately, there are three categories of difficulty that clearly overlap with each other (Fig 4.38).

Inability to give treatment enough priority

At an essentially practical level, some patients lead busy lives with many conflicting commitments. This can apply in all walks of life — home-makers, lawyers, physiotherapists and freelance artists have been amongst those falling into this category. While one appointment can be managed, setting up a series of appointments, and committing time to the programme in between visits proves too much. This becomes evident either from the start, or soon afterwards. For these busy people, an acceptance of living **with** eczema is a sacrifice they see they have to make, as otherwise other important arrangements in their life are jeopardised. If this involves employment or income, they will not see their skin condition as sufficiently important to risk creating problems in other arenas.

At one level, this is a dilemma for the individual to decide on. Things change and the programme can be used later with more benefit if it then suits the individual better. Thus treatment can be scheduled for a university student, or a school attender, to fit in with their vacation and holidays. It can be relevant however to emphasise how in the long term time is saved by successful treatment. The improved quality of life that comes has many knock-on effects, including improved efficiency and effectiveness, both with studies, and at work.

Inability to understand the programme

Because of personality attributes it sometimes becomes apparent that a patient is not suited to being helped in the particular way in which the programme is structured. Such difficulties are not necessarily a matter of intelligence, or emotional investment in illness. After a short time working with these patients it becomes clear they haven't taken in what has been discussed, and despite further explanation they are unable to carry out the new behaviours required. At the second visit the registration will not have been accomplished, the patient handbook or the tally-counter lost or left at home, and questions will be asked that demonstrate a failure to grasp what is involved. During the treatment phase, despite spoken and written instructions, all levels of treatment seem too much for the patient, and the basics for each level are not appreciated, even after repeated review. Some will listen attentively throughout, and appear to take in what is discussed, only to come back as if nothing has been learnt, and yet more is expected. Others will be over-talkative, and because of this nothing significant is gained from what is offered: the therapist will constantly have to interrupt the patient, in an attempt to cover the ground involved.

The approach we use is designed to suit most people, most of the time. For particular people, who can commit the time required and who genuinely want to be helped, it is necessary to try adapting the process involved to suit the individual. Some will simply need more time and patience, others will benefit from the involvement of a friend or relative. Particular problems will require imaginative solutions — the programme consists of a number of overlapping elements that allow for adaptation to personal needs.

Inability to give up chronic eczema

This is perhaps the most significant difficulty, and clearly it sometimes influences the first two problems discussed above. Summarised as an **emotional investment in illness**, it is evidently a phenomenon that can unfortunately complicate all types of long-standing disability. In atopic skin disease, over a period of years and beginning in childhood, the experience of the illness and its treatment becomes for some an essential and emotionally important part of day-to-day life. As atopic skin disease begins for many in the first year of life, causing sometimes understandable alarm and despondency in the parents, the child learns how relevant their condition can be in their relationship with the external world, and with their parents in particular. Before they are able to speak, they have a powerful means of gaining parental attention which can have long-standing effects in the development of their personality. For some to **live without eczema** is understandably a daunting prospect. This can be consciously appreciated and spontaneously referred to by some patients, while for others the issue will be buried from view, deep in their unconscious.

85

Tackling this problem may be relevant in the management of many patients, and fortunately a relatively straight-forward approach is successful for most. Explaining how the difficulty arises is usually easily accepted. Indeed, some will explain how the phenomenon is relevant for them, without any prompting from the therapist. For others the realisation that this difficulty is relevant will gradually emerge — first for the therapist, then for the patient. When this happens there is clearly a fertile opportunity for addressing the problem. Discussion in a here-and-now manner can be effective, especially if subsequent extra encouragement and support for appropriate behavioural change can be given. For others psychodynamic psychotherapeutic help, individually or in group therapy may be indicated. Such work will sometimes require a comprehensive and thorough process, but for others useful results can be achieved with a short-term approach focused on specific issues. Thus 'giving up illness' can be seen as a **grieving process**, with a need to 'work through' what is involved. During this process a **depressive reaction** can be understandable, both as something is being given up, and also because the years of illness that have been endured up to now will seem suddenly to have been so unnecessary.

Unfortunately there will remain some patients for whom insight into what is involved seems totally absent. Any suggestion that psychotherapy is worth considering is immediately placed out of court. The emotional resistance generated by the discussion can serve to confirm any initial suspicions on behalf of the therapist. It is evidently sensible not to pursue such difficult cases remorselessly, but to adopt a pragmatic approach. Agreeing that outcome has proved relatively unsuccessful so far, it will be appropriate to offer a review of the situation at a later date. As things change in the life of the individual, there may be opportunities for successful therapy later, even when previously all hopes of success seemed out of the question.

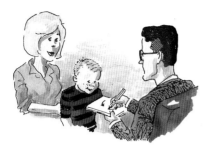

5

WORKING WITH YOUNGER CHILDREN

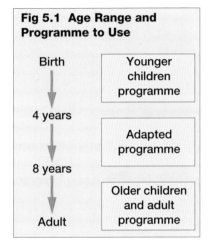

Fig 5.1 Age Range and Programme to Use

Birth	Younger children programme
4 years	Adapted programme
8 years	Older children and adult programme
Adult	

Fig 5.2 Key Messages

Parental awareness

=

Registration

•

Parents instructed in the three levels

•

Subsequent vigilance ensures success

5.1 Introduction

Age range

Although the programme for adults applies to children in their teens, and a similar approach is appropriate in older pre-teenage children, for younger children, infants and babies an adapted approach is required. Between the youngest patient and older children a programme can be constructed to suit the individual and their family (Fig 5.1).

Characteristics of work with the very young

Registration with the very young is unnecessary. For them, their parents are available to be aware of behaviour. Furthermore, it is the parents who need to understand the three levels of treatment, and who need to be instructed in how to deal with subsequent relapses through continuing awareness of the child's skin condition (Fig 5.2).

Stages in treatment

Once **chronic** atopic skin disease is established in the youngest patient by the vicious circle already described (p. 60), as in older patients a **change in behaviour** is required for healing to occur, as well as appropriate topical treatment. This change can usually be accomplished in days rather than weeks, i.e. a shorter period than in adulthood — though topical treatment is required for a similar period to that required in older patients. Once the vicious circle is broken and healing

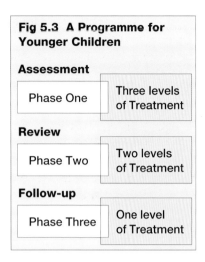

Fig 5.3 A Programme for Younger Children

Assessment

| Phase One | Three levels of Treatment |

Review

| Phase Two | Two levels of Treatment |

Follow-up

| Phase Three | One level of Treatment |

has been thoroughly accomplished, the follow-up period is again vital to prevent relapse into chronicity (Fig 5.3).

5.2 Assessment

History

Awareness (Fig 5.4)

As with older patients, history taking with younger children and their parents has both explicit and implicit functions. The explicit relevance of knowing about the current, recent and past condition of the skin, together with other associated medical, psychological and social factors, is evident. The process of this review can however serve also to heighten awareness for all concerned of the importance of behaviour, and appropriate attitudes towards atopic eczema and its treatment.

Behaviour

As set out in our suggested protocol (p. 111), a review of onset, distribution, and course is complemented by analysis of self-damaging behaviour. As well as clarifying how the condition has fluctuated, and listing the possible ameliorating and exacerbating external factors for future reference, the family is encouraged to remember and have listed the **situations, circumstances** and **activities** that are characteristically associated with scratching and rubbing. If time is made between the first visit and introducing treatment at a second visit, there will be an opportunity for the family to consider this further and discuss their observations on return. To clarify the relevance of this discussion, early use of the Handbook for Younger Children and their Parents is helpful (Appendix 3).

A few moments spent considering **how** the child scratches and rubs will prompt the family to consider that over time much of what has been happening may have been overlooked (Plate 5.1). A review of the **consequences** of scratching serves especially to highlight the social repercussions of self-damaging behaviour, and provides an early opportunity to consider simple issues in behaviour modification.

Fig 5.4 Key Messages

Assessment of the Younger Child

Facilitated by using handbook

•

Awareness increased by homework

•

Practical considerations relevant

•

Consider family attitudes and behaviour

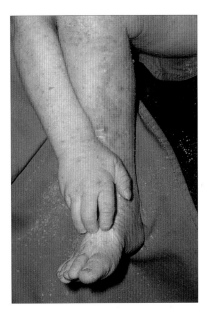

Plate 5.1   Scratching. A youngster with atopic eczema scratching his leg vigorously and shedding much skin onto the examination couch.

Social circumstances

Planning a programme with a family requires an appreciation of the current social arrangements at home. As with older patients, the successful application of The Combined Approach can be frustrated by practical considerations. With a full complement of willing and able family members to enlist for help, all will go well. Even a single parent of an only child can find others to involve successfully. However, when there are for example tensions between family members, these can be highlighted by the cooperation required in the first stage of treatment, and they will frustrate progress if they are not effectively addressed.

Background

Assessment includes a review of other illnesses. It may be important to note a history of food intolerance by enquiring about bowel habits. In family history it is particularly important to note any atopic skin disease in other family members, how successfully it has been treated and any clues as to the attitudes held regarding the illness and its management.

A review of development to date is clearly relevant for any child, but with atopic illness and its treatment it is particularly prudent to establish current developmental status, against which progress can be compared later if necessary.

Observation

Assessment is the first opportunity to observe directly both the patient, and the family. The success of the first interview can be made more likely by prior planning. Provision of appropriate distracting activities, and asking more than one family member to attend is useful. The condition of the skin is rated with the family, and the interaction between the child and others present is noted. The child's interest in the assessment is of particular relevance for all involved. Often during behavioural analysis it becomes clear that a child is not only engrossed in play, but is also listening carefully to what is being said. A parent's view can be suddenly corrected, or added to in such a way as to make the relevance of the discussion to the child only too apparent. This active involvement by the child in assessment is helpful in gauging the ability of the patient to be involved in treatment.

89

5.3 Treatment

Introduction

The patient handbook

As already mentioned, it is helpful to support treatment with previously prepared written material. In addition to the handbook it is useful to provide additional diagrams, instructions and information during consultations, to emphasise points relevant to each discussion.

The main principles of the treatment approach are as for older children and adults, and are dealt with in previous chapters. They will not therefore be repeated again in detail in this section, but they should nevertheless be considered for each patient and their family.

The protocol (Fig 5.5)

The number and frequency of visits required, together with the length of each visit and how the patient handbook is given to the family, can be varied according to circumstances. The younger the child and the larger the group interviewed, the more time needed. For example, for a child of two years with both mother and father, the first visit can take up to an hour and a half, but much less time **may** produce equally good results, especially when the therapist is experienced.

The first visit allows for assessment and explanation of the approach. A second visit can then be arranged to plan the treatment and the third visit will follow the first intensive phase of treatment. A further consultation is useful towards the end of the second phase, perhaps two or three weeks after starting treatment. Once the follow-up phase has started visits can be quite short and infrequent, but should be arranged prospectively to provide encouragement, support and continuing advice. All families find it helpful to have access to the therapist between visits, e.g. by telephone. During the first phase of treatment when activity at home is most intensive the therapist may telephone the family to give extra support, or a home visit may be appropriate, if practical to arrange.

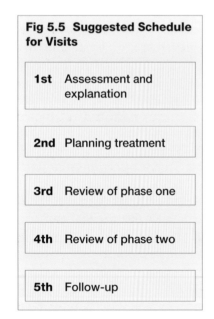

Fig 5.5 Suggested Schedule for Visits

1st	Assessment and explanation
2nd	Planning treatment
3rd	Review of phase one
4th	Review of phase two
5th	Follow-up

Phase 1: all three levels

Explaining the programme

From the beginning the distinction between long–standing atopic skin disease and recent relapses needs clarification.

Hence the importance of the vicious circle in demonstrating the **three** levels of treatment for chronic atopic eczema. The effort required by all concerned to break free from self-damaging behaviour must be acknowledged. Once this has been accomplished, the management of the condition becomes much easier. As the quality of life for the child and the family will immediately improve, with noticeable benefits for the child in many more aspects than skin alone, the hard work required can be seen to be not only time limited, but also an important investment. The months of misery that accompany the long-standing condition are replaced subsequently by episodes of illness that can be treated quickly and effectively in only a few days.

It is therefore vital that failure to deal with self-damaging scratching behaviour, coupled with inadequate use of conventional topical treatments are understood to be the two most significant causes of chronic atopic eczema (Fig 5.6).

Fig 5.6 Key Messages

The Common Causes of Chronic Eczema

Inadequate topical treatment

•

Self-damaging behaviours

The vicious circle of chronic eczema

Using the patient handbook and additional drawings and notes as necessary, the way in which the chronic syndrome develops is discussed. Although allergy is particularly relevant to hay fever and asthma, and has relevance in understanding atopic eczema, in the latter condition the **dryness** of the skin is of great practical significance. Both eczema and dryness lead to itch, while eczema and dryness relate to each other in a reciprocal manner.

The reciprocal relationship between itch and scratch is also important — though itch leads to scratch, scratch can lead to itch. In discussing this, the opportunity needs to be taken to clarify that **itching** is a **feeling:** it is not something that can be seen. In contrast **scratching** is a behaviour, an **action**; as such it can be observed. It then follows that itching and scratching are not to be confused and are not necessarily and irrevocably linked — each can occur without the other.

The experimental evidence of the effects of scratching (p. 44) should always be reviewed when explaining the operation of the vicious circle. The 'scratching machine' of the experiment is a useful concept to refer to, thus **turning off** the machine allows the latent healing processes in skin to assert themselves. That healing itself can be an itchy phenomenon needs to be appreciated.

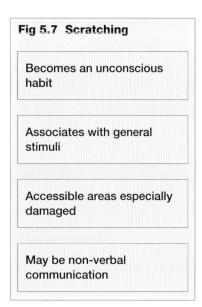

Fig 5.7 Scratching

Becomes an unconscious habit

Associates with general stimuli

Accessible areas especially damaged

May be non-verbal communication

Fig 5.8 Emollients: Questions to Answer

How do they work?

What is available?

When are they used?

For the child a reference to 'bees busy making honey' may be helpful, i.e. *'when you feel the buzzing of the bees, busy making honey, don't disturb them — else they'll get cross and no healing, or honey, will come'.*

If the child has been apparently engrossed in play or drawing up to this point in the interview, discussion of 'the scratching machine' and the effects of turning it off will often provoke a contribution from the patient.

It is clearly important to discuss how scratching is, over time, an increasingly habitual behaviour and as such all may have become relatively unaware of its occurrence (Fig 5.7). Although originally provoked by a particular stimulus, it tends later to generalise. Then it becomes linked to a variety of situations and circumstances, such as being bored or frustrated. The accessibility of skin for scratching, and the distribution of chronic eczema are important to review. The way scratching can become used, consciously or unconsciously, in family interpersonal communication is of particular importance. The testimony of some adult patients clearly endorses the notion that scratching for the child can be a powerful communication signal. That scratching can establish itself as a habit before the child can communicate through speech is clearly relevant. For the child, as for the adult, scratching can connect eczema to the rest of life.

Level 1: emollients (Fig 5.8)

Anyone treating a child should understand as much as possible about the treatment being used. It is relevant therefore to review with the parents the basis for drying of the skin in eczema (pp. 15–17) and to consider the phenomenon of constitutionally dry skin. How emollients correct dryness needs explanation, i.e. by moisturising **and** lubricating. The balance between body fluids and relative humidity of surrounding air helps explain how need for moisturising varies according to circumstances. How to apply emollients (p. 65) — thinly, gently, quickly and frequently — can then be understood, as can the principle that use of emollients is optimal as a **prevention** rather than a **treatment** of dry skin. The best results are achieved by anticipating that the skin will otherwise dry, and applying a fresh layer of moisturiser proactively.

The range of products available (Appendix 4) can be usefully considered, together with the different approaches to moisturising. The advantages and disadvantages of various creams and ointments, and the use of soap substitutes and bath additives can be included in this discussion to ensure maximum benefits are achieved.

The relationship between emollient use and the use of topical steroids should be mentioned. We recommend the application of an emollient on each occasion topical steroids are used, moisturising the skin over a wider area than that treated with topical steroid, and applying the emollient after the steroid, as a dressing. Neither application should be rubbed in as this action is unnecessary and can provoke itch. Both should therefore be wiped on, quickly and gently: **'only a shine is required'**.

Emollients are clearly to be used often during the day, usually on their own. Hence the rule: **topical steroids are never used on their own, emollients often are!**

Level 2: topical steroids (Fig 5.9)

In view of the particular sensitivity of children to steroid side-effects, there is an understandable and justified wariness of their use, especially in the earliest years. Parents need to understand that such side-effects are caused by inappropriate and misguided use. Used properly and under supervision, preferably with clear written instructions, topical steroids are the best pharmacological treatment for eczema and itch. They must be used for long enough, which can mean for several weeks when the condition has become chronic, and they must be strong enough, which means use of a potent steroid.

It is important to prevent parents from stopping the treatment when healing is only **cosmetic** — such healing is not long-lasting (p. 25). **Histological** healing must be the aim. When this is achieved there are **no subsequent immediate flare-ups** or relapses with discontinuation of topical steroid treatment.

Hence the key lesson for the concerned parent is that there is more risk of developing and maintaining chronic eczema with weak steroids, or too short a treatment period, than developing side-effects from a potent preparation. Less potency literally means less effectiveness; **good effects** must be the aim of treatment. They cannot be achieved if **side-effects** are an over–riding concern.

Unlike other approaches, The Combined Approach is effective because all common factors in chronic eczema are accounted for at the same time. Because self-damaging behaviour is reduced and eliminated, the topical

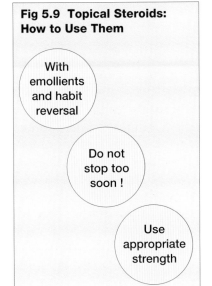

Fig 5.9 Topical Steroids: How to Use Them

With emollients and habit reversal

Do not stop too soon !

Use appropriate strength

steroids and emollients become a successful treatment. While there is no topical treatment strong enough to deal with the damage caused by scratching, habit reversal without proper use of topical steroids and moisturisers will not be effective. A **combined** approach is necessary.

Level 3: habit reversal (Fig 5.10)

As a behaviour modification technique based on learning theory, habit reversal (Ch 3) is usually of interest to parents. Time should be spent discussing behavioural analysis — the importance of antecedents and consequences, as well as the behaviour itself. Important principles need clarification, especially the need for **understanding** and **motivation**, and the significance of keeping all interventions **positive.** The child needs to know what to do, and not what not to do.

No habit can be successfully treated until **awareness** has been accomplished. In older children and adults preliminary registration by the patient is necessary. In the youngest patient the parents and others are available to observe behaviour and be aware of the situations most likely to be provocative. Parents will already be concerned about scratching, but they seldom appreciate the extent to which it is occurring, or understand the relevance of scratching in the development of chronic eczema. Explanation and instructions given by the therapist serve to make the family aware of the behaviour that needs modification. If time is allowed between first visit and starting treatment, an opportunity will be available for the family to make their own observations for further discussion.

As for adults, for children there are two types of scratching. There is scratching because of itching, and scratching because of circumstances. If the child is old enough to understand, **'itch scratch'** can be controlled without damaging the skin by teaching the child to pinch or press a fingernail into the itching area. The procedure needs to be actively demonstrated to both parents and child. If the child is able to participate in this way they gain an important sense of being **actively involved** in the healing process. Children as young as three years old have been taught how to use this method. After a week of treatment using The Combined Approach the procedure becomes redundant, as the behaviour of young children changes quickly.

Fig 5.10 Requirements for Changing Behaviour

- Understanding the old behaviour

- Motivation for change

- Knowing what to do

- Doing it !

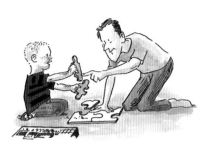

If the child is too young to participate in the way described, the following procedures designed in particular to tackle **'circumstance scratching'** will be sufficient for both types of self-damaging behaviour. The principles for dealing with this second type of scratching are therefore most important. First, successful and desirable behaviours need to be practised which are incompatible with the old, undesirable behaviour. Having agreed that rubbing and scratching the skin represents the latter, the family can draw up an inventory of safe behaviours in written form for all to refer to and add to as the treatment progresses. Inevitably **talk, play, diversion** and **distraction** are characteristic of all these desirable behaviours — and they should be **active**. Many will already be commonly practised, and imagination and suggestions from others will extend the list.

Next a review of the circumstances, activities and situations associated with scratching will reveal that some can be dispensed with for the time of the treatment programme, while others will prove unavoidable (Fig 5.11). Watching television alone should be avoided, while changing clothes is unavoidable. As with adults, the indispensable situations need to be adapted to limit or eliminate self-damaging behaviour. Planning ahead, keeping the hands busy, and doing things as quickly as possible are clearly useful tactics. Before changing clothes, all that is required needs to be assembled and the child given an interesting object to hold in both hands — preferably something soft! Then the change is accomplished purposefully and quickly. It is important when discussing this approach to emphasise that the method is only required for the time being. Everyone can relax once healing has been accomplished. Habit reversal is only required to break the vicious circle of chronic eczema.

These specific and general coping behaviours are underwritten by two most important instructions for successful habit reversal:

(a) never say *'Don't scratch!'*,
(b) never leave the child alone in the first four days of the treatment programme.

All successful interventions aimed at changing behaviour are couched in positive terms. **Negative entreaty** is to be avoided at all costs — saying *'don't'* is a recipe for encouraging a behaviour, not preventing it. We sum this up for families by teaching the slogan, *'Don''t* **Don't,** *Do* **Do!***'*.

Fig 5.11 Dealing with Difficult Circumstances

1. Have a plan

2. Do it quickly

3. Keep the hands busy

95

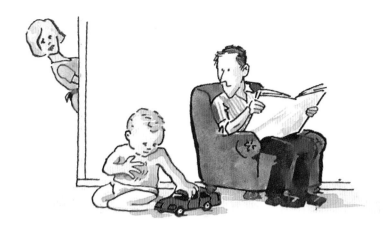

Secondly, as explained above, behavioural change requires awareness, and the parents and others who can be recruited to help are needed to achieve this awareness. During the first three or four days of intensive treatment the child is never to be left alone, not even for a second in difficult situations. This needs planning, as **supervision** is required day and night. It is useful for turns to be taken — a rota can be drawn up, and all involved need to understand the principles of what is required, and have available, as well as to contribute to, the list of suggestions for adaptive ways of coping with difficult situations. When the sleeping child is seen to be scratching, the watching adult gently takes the child from the bed and, holding the hands away from the skin, gives a hug and if necessary offers a distraction to calm and settle. As well as responding appropriately to difficult situations, it is equally if not more important for praise, support and encouragement to be given when scratching is not occurring, especially when the child is actively practising an adaptive response themselves.

In summary, there are 12 important rules for parents, six more general and six essentially practical (Fig 5.12).

Once the first three or four days have been successfully accomplished, the first phase of treatment continues with attention being applied especially to continuing treatment at Levels 1 and 2, emollients and topical steroids. Awareness of any self-damaging behaviour remains important and vigilance with continuing appropriate positive intervention is necessary, but gradually the intensity of this particular behavioural focus can lessen. As the skin heals the success of the treatment approach needs

Fig 5.12 Twelve Rules for Parents

General

1. Be aware of difficult situations

2. Prepare and plan ahead

3. Encourage: reward adaptive responses

4. Never say '*stop scratching*' — all intervention must be positive

5. **Active** talk, play, distraction and diversion

6. Follow all provocative activities and situations with a diversionary activity involving positive action

Practical

1. Avoid use of topical treatment less than 20 minutes before going to bed

2. Apply topical treatments quickly

3. Baths must be supervised

4. Pat the skin dry with a towel after washing

5. Undress and dress quickly

6. Sit with the child when watching television

reinforcement. Positive outcome is directly proportional to the effort applied at all three levels. By the end of the second week phase one will be overtaken by phase two — continuing treatment at Levels 1 and 2, to consolidate the progress achieved.

Phase two: Levels 1 and 2

The younger the child, the easier it is to modify behaviour. The healing process clearly benefits from an early cessation of scratching and rubbing, but a further finite period of time is needed to allow healing to be completed. A consultation during this phase ensures that topical treatment is continued appropriately, and in particular that the temptation to stop using topical steroids when the 'Look Good Point' (p. 67) is reached is not given in to.

This phase comes to an end when topical steroids are stopped. At this point the skin has appeared superficially healed for a week or more, and during the last few days of this phase the steroid used can be applied once daily, or a reduced potency steroid can be used twice a day. Those steroids that are used once daily at first, can now be applied on alternate days.

If an early relapse occurs, and becomes significantly complicated again by rubbing and scratching, it may be necessary to repeat the intensive programme of phase one.

However, if the relapse is associated with the end of topical steroid treatment, the most likely explanation is inadequate 'hidden healing'. The remedy then is to reinstitute treatment as soon as possible at Level 2, continuing Level 1 throughout. If the relapse is treated in this way further intensive treatment at Level 3 can be avoided.

5.4 Follow-up: Phase Three

Once healing has been thoroughly accomplished histologically, the most significant phase of management starts — follow-up. With the discontinuation of treatment at Levels 3 and 2, only emollient therapy at Level 1 continues. Eventually, unless the patient has constitutionally dry skin, even moisturisers may prove unnecessary.

The first two stages of healing of chronic eczema, cosmetic or **obvious**, which is superficial, and histological or **hidden**, which is deeper and involves the resolution of all inflammatory processes in the superficial dermis, is followed by two or three months when

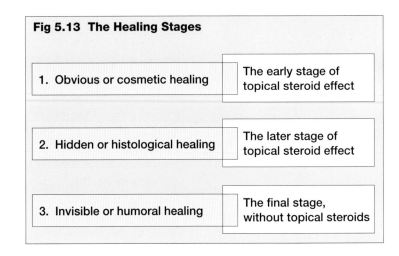

Fig 5.13 The Healing Stages

1. Obvious or cosmetic healing	The early stage of topical steroid effect
2. Hidden or histological healing	The later stage of topical steroid effect
3. Invisible or humoral healing	The final stage, without topical steroids

humoral rather than histological or structural changes occur. This extended convalescence can be called **invisible healing**. As this last phase progresses the natural resilience of the skin returns, and some if not all of the hypersensitivities that can characterise eczematous skin will disappear (Fig 5.13).

During follow-up, **vigilance** by the parents is most important. This applies even if, with the return of normal skin, emollients have been discontinued. Every day the skin needs inspection for signs of relapse and when diagnosed treatment should be started again immediately (Fig 5.14). In order to emphasise the importance of this prompt response the slogan,

'Zap the Relapse'

is used, and each patient should have the necessary treatment available: the **Zap Pack**.

For any relapse an effective topical steroid needs to be used for at least six days, for example **three days twice daily**, **three days once daily**, with the **Look Good Point** on day two, or three. If this point takes longer to achieve, the treatment period needs extending: the period taken for 'hidden healing' can be approximately equal the time taken for 'obvious healing'. Thus, treatment of an acute relapse, if started early and pursued vigorously, will be successful in a matter of days, rather than the weeks needed for chronic eczema.

With the topical steroid, emollient therapy is essential, and initially is required frequently. Once healing has occurred moisturisers will be necessary for at least a week or two longer, if not more, depending on both skin and environmental factors.

By returning to the experiences recorded at first assessment, discussion can usefully focus on the factors known to provoke eczematous reactions. Some of these will be **given** and therefore unavoidable. Some will be **intermittent** and variable. Atopy itself is a given vulnerability factor which cannot be avoided. Seasonal changes are usually unavoidable. Intermittent factors include other climatic variations, episodes of stress and unhappiness, and periods of physical strain and exhaustion including perhaps concomitant physical illnesses (Fig 5.15). Parents can appreciate that when several factors occur together a relapse is more likely, and action can be taken. It may be possible to change arrangements to offset the possibility of a relapse. Emollient treatment can be reinstated, or

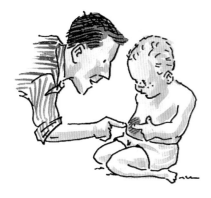

Fig 5.14 Relapse Recognition

- Dryness

- Roughness

- Redness

- Itchiness

Fig 5.15 Vulnerability and Provocative Factors

Unavoidable	Avoidable
• Atopy	• Exhaustion
• Season	• Stress
• Climate	• Air conditioning
• Illness	• Allergies

given more often. Vigilance becomes even more important, in order that any relapse which proves unavoidable can be treated early and vigorously. Hence a further slogan for parents: *'Help stamp out chronic eczema!'*.

It is evident that managing the skin condition successfully in this way is worth accomplishing. The relatively continuous experience of skin disease in the chronic condition is replaced by intermittent episodes of acute relapse (p. 83). As these are managed appropriately they become less troublesome and less frequent as convalescence progresses. Now the skin is being managed by the family rather than the family being managed by the skin. They are living **without**, rather than **with** eczema.

5.5 Problems

As in adulthood

The three main types of difficulty preventing successful treatment of adults (p. 84, Fig 4.38) can be seen in their own form in young children and their families. Thus for families the practicalities of The Combined Approach for the very young patient can compete unsuccessfully with other priorities and considerations. Evidently the first phase of intensive treatment requires time and effort, and this needs commitment. Hopefully this is worthwhile for the majority of families, but this will not always be the case.

Secondly, the ability of those involved to understand what is required will vary. The instructions can sometimes seem difficult for an individual parent to absorb. This becomes evident when the programme has not been followed, and review reveals that essential principles have not been appreciated.

Often ways round these practical and educational problems can be found. More difficult for the younger child are the equivalents to the attitudinal problems of adulthood, and it is particularly in the adults of the family where these issues will be encountered. They range from an impervious resistance to using topical steroids properly, to an evident emotional investment in continuing illness. With the latter case, rarely and at its most extreme the situation for the child resembles an **illness by proxy.** Without the child continuing to need treatment, the parent would not have access to health centres and hospitals. Once recognised as a significant problem, the focus of concern must be moved from the child to the parent. The emotional needs of the adult need to be investigated, understood and adaptively met before care of the child can be successful.

Eczema in both child and parent

A particularly striking difficulty occasionally encountered is when both young child and a parent has troublesome atopic skin disease, yet it is the child that is presented as the patient. The parent who has suffered with eczema themselves since childhood and on into adulthood carried a burden of frustration and unhappiness that, together with specific beliefs about eczema and its treatment, unavoidably influences the care of the child. Once we recognised this important phenomenon, we have regularly asked when a child comes for assessment if either parent has active atopic skin disease. Incidentally it has also now become of interest to ask all adult patients if as children they were treated at home by a parent who had themselves had atopic eczema, or if now as adults they have a child or children at home with eczema.

If a parent of a child brought for assessment with atopic eczema also has active eczema, there is a strong case for treating the parent first, as set out in Chapter 4. In this way they can learn the principles of The Combined Approach at first hand, and will become in the process much more positive and effective in the management of their child's disease.

The immune status of the child

In the earliest months of life, when atopic skin disease can first manifest itself, The Combined Approach as described above applies as it does for the toddler and the young infant. The healing response in these very young patients can be unpredictable however, as the immature immune system seems to fluctuate in its effectiveness, sometimes frustrating the very best treatment approach. This possibility should be considered when the programme is started with a child under 12 months; a disappointing early relapse can then be accommodated without giving up on The Combined Approach altogether. With some months further maturity the

**Fig 5.16 Why Some Young
Children do Less Well**

- Treatment low priority

- Programme not understood

- Unhelpful attitudes

- Immature immune system

- Hyperallergic syndrome

immune response becomes more predictable, and healing sustained following conscientious treatment.

Apart from immaturity affecting immune status, as for adults (p. 83), in childhood there are unfortunately examples of profound constitutional hypersensitivity to environmental factors. Such hyperallergic children are not commonly encountered, but when met they pose very serious difficulties for any treatment programme. The Combined Approach will clearly be important as it offers a very relevant treatment package. The results however will be less than optimal, as for this small group of unhappy children some degree of chronic illness is difficult to avoid (Fig 5.16).

6

CONCLUSIONS

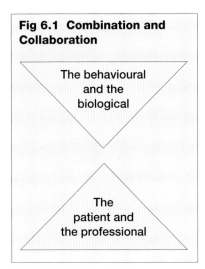

Fig 6.1 Combination and Collaboration

The behavioural and the biological

The patient and the professional

6.1 Final conversations

The approach to atopic skin disease described in this manual combines behavioural psychotherapy techniques with dermatological treatment. However, there is also another important combination, that of the **professional's expertise** and the **patient's experience**. The development of The Combined Approach owes much to the observations and ideas of people with atopic skin disease who have been our patients. The importance of this **collaboration** is often highlighted in the final conversation with a patient, before discharge from the clinic (Fig 6.1).

The successful treatment of chronic eczema can bring with it a new lease of life, characterised by a sense of increased freedom and dramatically improved self-confidence. The improvements in quality of life are striking, and serve to underline the hidden unhappiness that almost invariably comes with long-standing atopic skin disease. The delight that accompanies successful treatment is sometimes however tinged with regret. There is a sense of loss associated with the realisation that if the condition had been treated successfully sooner, much suffering could have been avoided.

Linked with this regret is an amazement that it has taken so long for the separate strands of the treatment to be brought together into one coordinated programme. In particular, patients are surprised how helpful it is to know more about their own condition, and the basic principles behind effective treatment. Thus they ask why no-one has previously taken the trouble to explain to them, for example, how emollients and topical steroids are believed to work.

103

Fig 6.2 Changing Habits

- Patient becomes a manager, rather than a victim

- Professional becomes an enabler, rather than a prescriber

6.2 Misconceptions about The Combined Approach

One purpose of providing others with our ideas in the form of this manual has been to correct frequent misconceptions about what is involved. It will be seen that The Combined Approach is not **just** 'habit reversal', i.e. the effective elimination of habitual self-damaging behaviours. Rather, the programme is an exercise in **behavioural medicine**, and uses many ideas borrowed from **cognitive behaviour therapy**. Any optimally successful treatment in medicine requires account to be taken of the relevant attitudes and behaviour of the patient, and this requirement is only met by the professional having appropriate attitudes, and behaving accordingly.

The 'habit reversal' that is involved is as much a change in the behaviour of the professional, as it is in the patient. The programme aims to **eliminate bad habits** by **establishing good habits** in their place.

The patient becomes a manager of their condition, rather than a victim of it, while the professional learns to enable this effective management by providing appropriate information, support and encouragement, as well as the traditional resource of correct medical treatment (Fig 6.2).

6.3 Promulgation of The Combined Approach

A further intention in writing this manual has been to make our experience more generally available. We hope that nurses and doctors in primary health care can begin to use the approach, together with those in hospital practice. The opportunities that exist for cross-fertilization of experience and expertise between general practice and hospital-based dermatology are clearly relevant. At first sight it may seem that the approach requires significant resources in terms of clinical time. We hope this is not the case. The aim of our programme is to eliminate a chronic and disabling condition, thereby releasing resources for other purposes. Thus the initial investment of time and energy is, in our experience, amply rewarded by the results (Fig 6.3).

Fig 6.3 Key Message

The elimination of chronicity saves time!

PROTOCOL FOR THE COMBINED APPROACH ('HABIT REVERSAL') TO ATOPIC SKIN DISEASE IN ADULTS AND OLDER CHILDREN

As Used at Daniel Turner Department of Dermatology, Chelsea & Westminster Hospital, London

Prior to the first visit for The Combined Approach, the patient is referred to the Department usually by the general practitioner, and seen by a dermatologist for assessment and diagnosis. A referral is then made to the Psychodermatology Service and a series of appointments is arranged.

Visit One

Introduction

Therapist introduced. Broad characteristics of programme described. Usual experience of treatment to date summarised — in contrast, The Combined Approach characterised by active involvement, with good reason for optimism. Emphasis to be on 'managing eczema' rather than 'being managed'.

Demography

Age, Employment, Marital Status and Dependents.

History of presenting complaint

Overview: until recently
* Since when?
* Then, which parts? How bad?

- Who treated? Did they have eczema?
- Asthma? Hayfever?
- Hospitalisation? Specialists?
- Quality of life effects: at home ? At school? Otherwise?
- Course of disease since origin till recently? Ever cleared?
- Any profound change in distribution or nature? When? How?

Now

- Fluctuations: better for days, weeks or months? Worse for days, weeks or months?
- Ever clears 100%? Quality of life effects?
- Recent use of topical treatment: Continuous? Intermittent?
- Factors worsening or improving: consider — stress, season, climate, work, home life, holidays, exercise, temperature, alcohol, menses, central heating, air conditioning, diet, animals, dust, weather, relationships.

Current state

1. Overall subjective severity on scale 0–10 (10 the worst ever, 0 perfect skin).
2. Percentage of eczema old vs. new eczema (new: in last few days — explain with graph showing fluctuating long–term disease and acute relapses).
3. Where mostly? Where otherwise?
4. Percentage of scratching coming from itch.

Current treatment

1. Emollients: Thinner? Thicker? Soap substitute? Bath or shower additive?
2. Topical steroids: For face? For body? For scalp?
3. Other treatments: Antihistamines? Systemic treatments? Treatment for other conditions? Psychotropic medication?

Behavioural analysis: antecedents

A typical day: situations, circumstances and activities associated with, or not associated with scratching, (with or without itching).

Introduce part one patient handbook

- Atopy.
- Relevance of scratching.
- The vicious circle.

- The three levels of treatment.
- Scratching and registration.

End of first visit

- Advise continue current treatment otherwise.
- Advise return for second visit with Part One handbook and tally-counter.

Visit Two

Review

- Check brought Part One handbook? Tally-counter?
- Record:
    1. Scratching frequencies per day.
    2. When scratching mostly.
    3. Percentage scratching from itch.
    4. Subjective 0–10 severity.
    5. Percentage new vs. old.
    6. Where mostly, and otherwise.

Behavioural Analysis:

How?
1. Nails?
2. Skin-on-skin rub?
3. Rubbing through clothing/use of towelling, etc.?
4. Rubbing against immovable objects?
5. Use of movable instruments?
6. Involving other persons?
7. Other methods scratching/rubbing, e.g. hot, or cold water? Use of teeth, use of stubble?

Consequences
1 Physical.
2 Emotional.
3 Social (especially significant others).

Background history

- General health: physical, psychological.
- Recent/current life events and social factors.
- Past history, especially chronic illness, allergies.
- Family history, especially atopy, relationship with parents.

- Personal history, especially education, psychosexual adjustment and marriage, children.
- Personality, especially interests, confidence, expressiveness and obsessiveness.

Objective findings

Physical
Skin, other systems.

Mental
Especially attitude, intelligence, personality, rapport.

Other procedures

- Photograph?
- Laboratory investigations?

Prognosis

Score out of 10 (10 the best) — give reasons.

Part two programme from patient handbook

1. The vicious circle.
2. The three levels of treatment.
3. Level 1: emollient treatment — principles of, instructions how.
4. Level 2: topical steroid treatment — principles of, instructions how.
5. Level 3: habit reversal — principles of behavioural change, specific measures, general measures, self–prescription for new behaviours.

Final advice visit two

- Prescriptions for Levels 1 and 2: written out in patient handbook.
- Instruct continuous registration.

Visit Three

Review

1. Registration of scratching frequency.
2. When mostly?

3. Percentage scratching from itch.
4. 0–10 severity?
5. Where mostly? Where otherwise?
6. Percentage old vs. new.

Three levels of treatment review

Level 1: Emollients.
Level 2: Steroids — check use of booklet.
Level 3: Habit reversal — specific measures, any adaptions introduced, general measures.

Review rationale — check understanding, answer questions

Review day and night behaviour, using 12 hour clock faces — draw diagrams and indicate by shading-in when patient 'most at risk'. Discuss strategies for focal attention in next period of home treatment. Demonstrate small proportion of day equals most damage done. Establish target frequency for scratching to be achieved by next visit.

'The healing curve'

Use graph drawn with patient to illustrate 'healing curve' compared with fluctuating chronic atopic skin disease — show three levels of treatment produce 'healing curve': emphasise all levels require active patient participation.

Trouble shooting

• Is stress significant factor? Review methods of coping — give written suggestions.
• Forgotten areas, e.g. scalp?
• Infections?
• Sensitivities?

End of third visit

• Review continuing treatment instructions.
• Replenish record sheets as necessary.

Visit Four

• Review 6 measures (see beginning of third visit).
• Review three levels of treatment (see third visit).

- Review usefulness of focal attention worked out in third visit.
- Consider 'three dimensions':
  1. Relevance of stress, and techniques of coping.
  2. Attitudes to illness before, and now.
  3. Attitudes to illness, from others.

- Review follow-up procedures:
  1. Graph of healing curve with three levels of treatment: show how treatments are discontinued sequentially. Review of importance relapse recognition. List symptoms and signs of relapse.
  2. Discuss reasons for relapse. Discuss relevance of 'continuous' compared with 'intermittent' causes of relapse.
  3. Give instructions for treatment of relapse — refer to vicious circle and Levels 1 and 2 — explain level 3 usually unnecessary.
  4. Remind principles emollients and topical steroid treatment.
  5. Discuss 'convalescent phase': increasing resilience of skin.
  6. Emphasise importance of continuous vigilance for relapse — versus discontinuing steroids, discontinuing emollients.
  7. Review need for skin to heal completely: ensure standards appropriate.

Subsequent Visits

- Review six measures (see third visit).
- Review progress since last visit — has skin cleared? For how long?
- Review signs of relapse.
- Review use of emollients.
- Review use of steroids.
- Review relevance of habit reversal.
- Review quality of life.
- Review stress management, attitudes of self, attitudes of others.
- Consider future strategies: ensure availability of Zap Pack for relapses.
- Discuss follow-up arrangements — further contacts.

PROTOCOL FOR THE COMBINED APPROACH ('HABIT REVERSAL') TO ATOPIC SKIN DISEASE IN YOUNGER CHILDREN

As Used at Daniel Turner Department of Dermatology, Chelsea & Westminster Hospital London

Prior to the first visit for The Combined Approach, the patient and parents are referred to the Department usually by the general practitioner, and seen by a dermatologist for assessment and diagnosis. A referral is then made to the Psychodermatology Service and a series of appointments is arranged.

Visit One

Introduction

Therapist introduced. Note who attends with child. Arrange distracting activity for child. Broad characteristics of programme described. Usual experience of treatment to date summarised — in contrast, The Combined Approach characterised by collaboration between family and therapist. Emphasis to be on 'managing eczema' rather than 'being managed'; education, by discussion and reading.

Demography

Age, other family members.

History of presenting complaint

Overview: until recently
- Since when?
- Then, which parts? How bad?
- Anyone else affected?
- Asthma? Hayfever?
- Hospitalisation? Specialists?

111

- Quality of life effects : at home ? At school? Otherwise?
- Course of disease since origin till recently? Ever cleared?
- Any profound change in distribution or nature? When? How?

Now
- Fluctuations: better for days, weeks or months? Worse for days, weeks or months?
- Ever clears 100%? Quality of life effects?
- Recent use of topical treatment: Continuous? Intermittent?
- Factors worsening or improving: consider — season, climate, home life, holidays, play, temperature, central heating, air conditioning, diet, animals, dust, weather, stress

Current state
1. Overall severity (parents' view) on scale 0–10 (10 the worst ever, 0 perfect skin).
2. Percentage of eczema old vs. new eczema (new: in last few days — explain with graph showing fluctuating long–term disease and acute relapses).
3. Where mostly? Where otherwise?
4. Evidence for 'habit–scratching' and 'circumstance–scratching'.

Current treatment
1. Emollients: Thinner? Thicker? Soap substitute? Bath or shower additive?
2. Topical steroids: For face? For body? For scalp?
3. Other treatments: Antihistamines? Systemic treatments? Treatment for other conditions?

Background history

- General health otherwise.
- Recent/current life events, social factors.
- Past history, especially chronic illness, allergies.
- Family history, especially atopy, relationship with parents.
- Developmental history: milestones.
- Personality.

Behavioural analysis: antecedents
A typical day: situations, circumstances and activities associated with, or not associated with scratching.

Objective findings

Physical
Skin, other systems.

Mental
Behaviour during consultation; relationship with parents

Other procedures

- Photograph?
- Laboratory investigations?

Prognosis

Score out of 10 (10 the best) — give reasons.

Introduce part one patient handbook

- Atopy.
- Relevance of scratching.
- The vicious circle.
- The three levels of treatment.
- Food, infections and clothing.
- Scratching: awareness.

End of first visit

- Advise continue current treatment otherwise.
- Advise return for second visit with Part One handbook and list of circumstances most associated with scratching.
- Explain practical aspects of Phase One, especially Level 3.

Visit Two

Review

- Check brought Part One handbook?
- Record:
  1. When scratching mostly.
  2. Percentage scratching due to habit or circumstance.
  3. 0–10 severity (parents' view).
  4. Percentage new vs. old.
  5. Where mostly, and otherwise.

How?

1. Nails?
2. Skin-on-skin rub?
3. Rubbing through clothing/use of towelling, etc.?
4. Rubbing against immovable objects?
5. Use of movable instruments?
6. Involving others?
7. Other methods?

Consequences

1. Physical
2. Emotional
3. Social (especially significant others)

- The vicious circle.
- The three levels of treatment.
- Level 1: emollient treatment — principles of, instructions how.
- Level 2: topical steroid treatment — principles of, instructions how.
- The use of creams.
- Level 3: habit reversal — habits, principles behavioural change, specific measures: scratching because of itch, general measures: scratching because of circumstances.
- Review of the programme, especially Phase One.
- Important rules and practical tips.

- Prescriptions for Levels 1 and 2 : written out in patient handbook.
- Level 3: difficult times and ways of coping. Arrangements for the first three or four days.

Visit Three

Any eczema remaining? If so

1. 0–10 severity?
2. Where mostly? Where otherwise?

3. Percentage old vs. new.
4. Circumstances associated with most scratching.

If no eczema visible
When was Look Good Point?

Three levels of treatment review

Level 1:   Emollients.
Level 2:   Steroids : check use of booklet.
Level 3:   Habit reversal — specific measures, any adaptions introduced. General measures.

> **Review rationale — check understanding, answer questions**

PLAN completion of Phase Two, as necessary

Part three programme from patient handbook

Phase three: follow–up

- Review Level 1
- Diagnosis of relapses.
- Treatment of relapses: provide schedule.
- Provide prescription.
- Arrange follow–up.

Subsequent visits

- Review progress.
- Clarify treatment plan: tailor to needs.
- Trouble shooting: forgotten areas? infections? hyper-sensitivities?
- Review reasons for relapses.
- Review quality of life, development.
- Discharge to primary care

LIVE WITHOUT ECZEMA

The Handbook for Adults and Older Children*

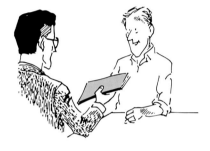

Part 1 Introduction

This approach to the treatment of atopic skin disease is **complementary** rather than **alternative** to conventional treatment. Existing treatment principles are added to, creating a programme that is very effective.

An important aspect of the programme is **behaviour modification** to eliminate the damage caused to skin by scratching. Also emphasised is the relevance of attitude and circumstance.

Chronic eczema causes **months and years of misery.** Let's replace all that with only the **days of inconvenience** needed for the effective treatment of acute relapses.

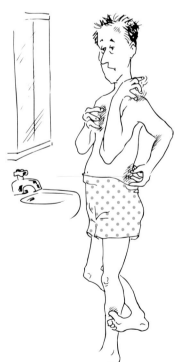

Atopy

Having 'atopy' means being born prone to develop eczema, hay fever and asthma. Hay fever and asthma are allergic conditions, like the rhinitis that is caused in summer by a high pollen count. Eczema is much more to do with dry skin.

---

*Not for photocopying. Further copies of this handbook can be obtained from the Publisher.

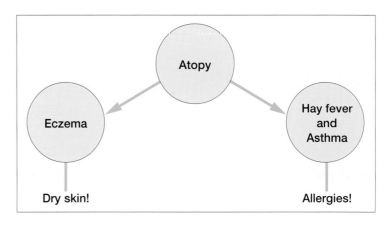

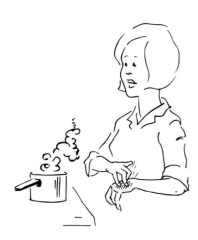

Dry skin tends to be itchy: this leads to scratching...

Scratching

Even normal skin when scratched will eventually look like chronic eczema under a microscope.

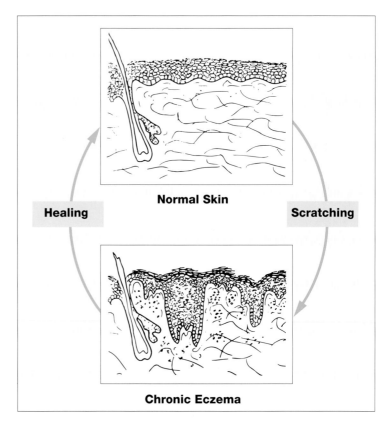

Normal Skin

Healing

Scratching

Chronic Eczema

Healing can only occur if scratching stops

So ...

With dryness, itching and scratching a vicious circle is established:

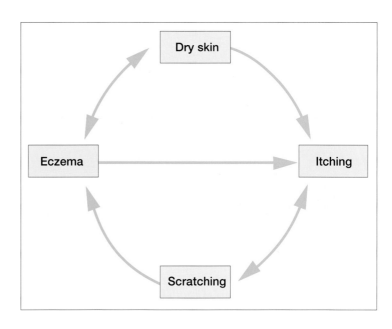

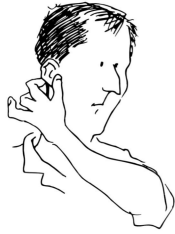

Areas that are easiest to scratch and rub are especially susceptible to chronic eczema.

Breaking the Vicious Circle

The vicious circle of chronic eczema has three levels

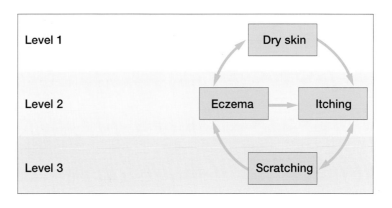

Conventional treatment provides emollients for Level 1 and topical steroids for Level 2... but **neither are sufficient for Level 3!**

Level 3 needs its own special treatment.

Chronic eczema only heals with all three levels of treatment, as described in The Programme ...

First, what about scratching?

1.   Scratching means **all** touching of the skin.

> **Scratching = Picking = Rubbing = Touching**

Scratching is the fastest and most effective way of getting relief from itch, but with atopic eczema the result is disastrous.

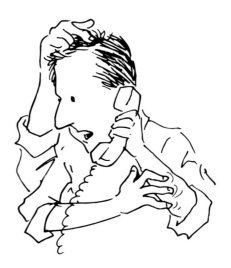

2.   Scratching in the beginning is a conscious reaction to itch. Later it becomes **habitual** and **unconscious**.

3.   Scratching begins as a behaviour stimulated by itch. Over time it becomes linked to other stimuli — it **generalises**.

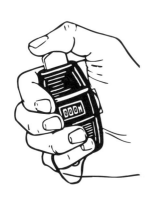

So, What Do We Do?....

Registration

As a habit becomes part of normal life, we grow unaware of it. One way of becoming aware of a habit is to measure its frequency, for example with the help of a hand-counter.

With each episode of scratching the counter is pressed. Each evening the result is registered on the chart provided. Registration is very important as it interferes with daily life, introduces discipline that is necessary for success and provides a result that can be easily measured.

The trouble taken in registration is the price to be paid for breaking the habit. Consistency and discipline for sufficient length of time are required for healing to occur.

Level 3 of treatment begins with registration, in order to map your behaviour.

> *Don't avoid scratching.*
> *Allow registration to make you more*
> *aware of your habit!*

REGISTRATION CHART

Name: _____ Date _____

Date							
Frequency of scratching							

*Scratching means **all** touching of the skin*

Scratching = Picking = Rubbing = Touching

**Don't avoid scratching.
Allow registration to make you more
aware of your habit!**

Make a note of your particularly scratchy situations:

1. _____

2. _____

3. _____

4. _____

Part 2: The Programme

The three levels of treatment

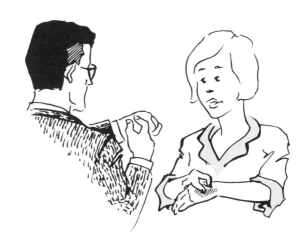

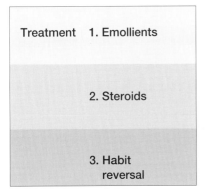

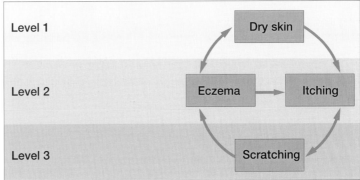

Level 1
The dry skin should be treated **consistently**, so that it never becomes dry. This is especially important with eczema on the face and neck.

Level 2
Eczema and itch should be treated **aggressively** with steroids.

Level 3
Scratching is treated with **discipline**.

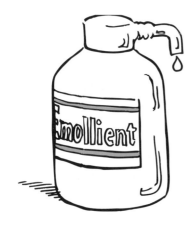

Level 1: Emollients

Atopic skin becomes dry because it is abnormally porous.

Dry skin must be treated with emollient, which prevents water loss and lubricates the skin. It is especially important to use emollients frequently at the beginning of treatment. The more inflamed, thickened and dry the skin is the more often an emollient must be used.

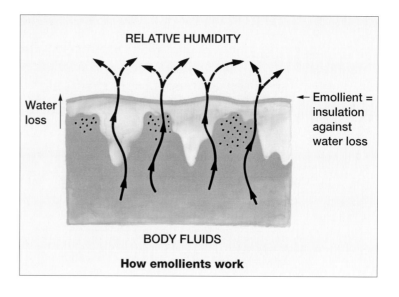

How emollients work

Use Emollients ...

- *Thinly*
- *Gently*
- *Quickly*
- *Frequently*

The drying of the skin will be affected by changes in the environment, and bodily function — know when more emollients will be needed!

Level 2: Steroids

Eczema and itch are effectively treated by steroid creams and ointments. The stronger the steroid the more effective it is. Fear of side-effects often results in inadequate treatment, with frequent and rapid relapses. Side-effects are not seen until after MANY weeks of treatment with strong steroids. There is more risk of developing **chronic** eczema with weak steroids, or with too short a treatment period, than of developing side effects from strong steroids.

How topical steroids work

The healing with topical steroids is in two stages. When the skin first looks good there is still some hidden healing to accomplish:

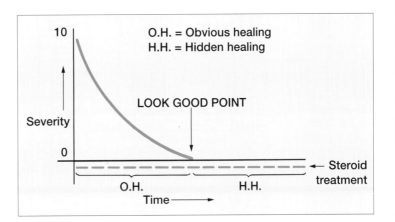

Use Steroids ...

- *As prescribed !*
- *Don't stop too soon !*

The use of creams

- All topical treatments must be used consistently — in a **planned** way. The application must be brisk and without any unnecessary massage. The steroid should be applied morning and/or evening, and the emollients are used as often as is necessary to prevent the skin from drying.

- The amount of cream that is used depends upon the area treated and how dry the skin is. After treatment the skin should not feel sticky ... **only a shine is required !**

- Apply the steroid on all areas affected by eczema.

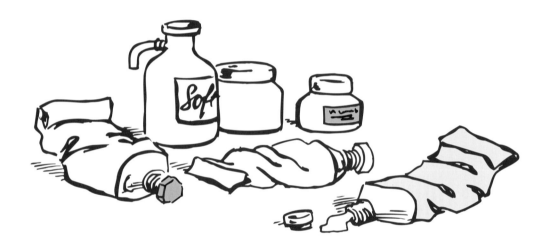

- Then emollient can be put over the whole body, and should be put on again as soon as the skin **begins** to dry. At the beginning of a treatment this could mean one hour after the steroid has been used — later on only once or twice a day.

- Emollients are thus used on areas treated and not treated with steroids. No steroid without emollients, but emollient can be used without steroid.

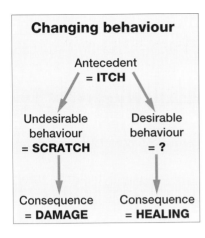

Changing behaviour

Antecedent = ITCH

Undesirable behaviour = SCRATCH

Desirable behaviour = ?

Consequence = DAMAGE

Consequence = HEALING

Level 3: Scratching

How do we change behaviour?

If the *antecedent* of an *undesirable behaviour* is followed instead by a *new behaviour* that is **incompatible** with the *old behaviour*, the *undesirable consequences* of the old behaviour will be avoided. The new and *desirable consequences* then reinforce and establish the new behaviour.

Habit reversal is the name given to the technique that we will use to change your behaviour ...

Old behaviour	New behaviour
(a) Automatic movement towards the itching area	(a) Squeeze your fist 30 seconds
(b) Scratching	(b) Pinch or press a nail into the part that itches

To begin with, practise the following several times daily:

1. Squeeze your fists moderately hard for 30 seconds, while thinking hard about any pleasing activity or event.

2. Relax a couple of seconds.

3. Choose a place which often itches.

4. Pinch or press a nail into the chosen spot for about 30 seconds.

> *From now on replace all scratching*
> *behaviour with your new habit.*
>
> *If there is no itch after fist-clenching*
> *there is no need to pinch.*

Situations which provoke scratching

List these situations and consider if any are **dispensable** for the next four weeks. If some can be dispensed with, scratching frequency will immediately decrease.

For situations which are **indispensable**, or when the **habit reversal** technique is difficult to use, introduce **damage limitation** tactics.

Damaging	Damage limitation
Scratching after a shower or bath	Pat the skin dry with a towel, put on the emollient, dress quickly and distract yourself for about 10 minutes
Scratching in bed	Get up!
Scratching while undressing	Be mentally prepared and undress quickly. Use your cream, dress again, then distract yourself for 10 minutes
Scratching while watching TV, talking on the phone, etc.	Keep your hands occupied!

If you have difficulties in remembering not to scratch, put up a sign e.g. on the bathroom door, on the TV, or by the phone.

> *Prepare yourself for difficult situations ...*
> *Anticipate and plan your own strategies!*

TREATMENT SCHEDULE

Name: _____ Date _____

Level 1: Emollients _____
_____
_____

Should be used: _____
_____
_____

Be consistent !

Level 2: Topical steroids

Date							
a.m.							
p.m.							

Date							
a.m.							
p.m.							

**Keep to the schedule —
don't stop too soon !**

Level 3: Habit reversal

Continue registration to measure your progress:

Date							
No of scratchings							

Date							
No of scratchings							

Date							
No of scratchings							

Date							
No of scratchings							

> **Prepare yourself!**
> **Do it quickly!**
> **Keep hands busy!**

Difficult situations

Dispense with:

1. _____
2. _____
3. _____
4. _____

Otherwise — keep to the following:

1. _____
2. _____
3. _____
4. _____

> **Success depends on your own efforts**

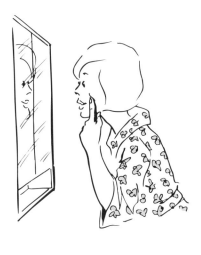

Part 3: Follow–up

- The three levels of treatment needed for long-standing atopic skin disease become unnecessary as the skin heals completely

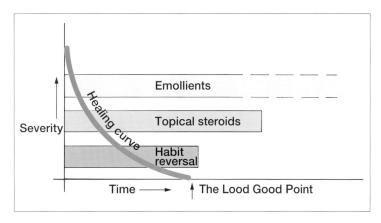

- The fluctuations in the severity of long-standing atopic eczema are now replaced by only short episodes of relapse

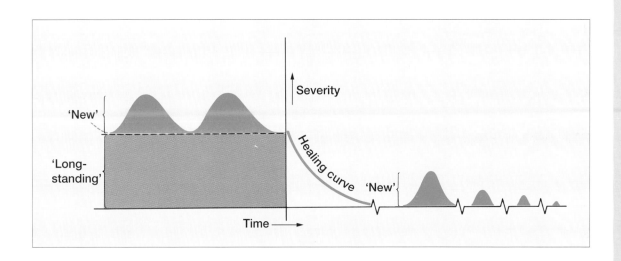

Once healing has been thoroughly accomplished, continue with Level 1 treatment only, as necessary — but beware of relapses!

LOOK at, and **FEEL** the skin daily during convalescence. Recently healed chronic eczema remains unstable for several weeks ...

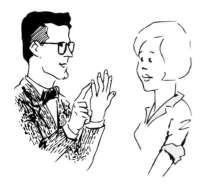

> ### *Think of ...*
>
> * *Itchiness*
> * *Dryness*
> * *Redness*
> * *Roughness*

When an acute relapse is identified — **TREAT IT !**

Help **STAMP OUT** chronic eczema ...

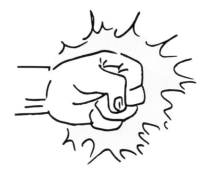

ZAP THE RELAPSE !

Remember !

Itch will go if relapse is treated promptly.

Regime for acute relapse

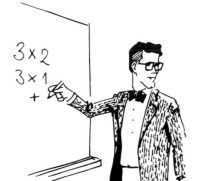

> ### *3 days steroid twice daily**
> ### *3 days steroid once daily*
> *plus*
> ### *Intensive use of emollients*
>
> * Topical steroids which are used once daily can subsequently be used on alternate days.

N.B.

> *There is no need to*
> **'Live with eczema'** ...
>
> *The aim of treatment is to*
> **'LIVE WITHOUT ECZEMA'** !

As convalescence progresses the skin becomes more stable ...

> ***Stop using emollients routinely!***
> ***Begin to assess the skin routinely!***

Look at the skin:

Is there redness, is it dry, rough or itchy?

- The more cautious you are
- The sooner you begin your treatment
- The stronger steroid you use
- The more consistent you are with emollients at the beginning of treatment

Then ...

- The sooner the skin will heal
- The less steroid will be used
- The less trouble you will get with eczema, and with side effects from both eczema and steroids

> **Remember !**
> *Consistent* use of emollients!
> ***Aggressive* use of steroids!**
> *Disciplined* behaviour!

Then there is only the predisposition to eczema to live with.

FOLLOW-UP SCHEDULE

Name: _____   Date _____

(A) Every day check for

Redness
Dryness
Itchiness
Roughness

(B) For any relapse treat with

Level 1: Emollients

_____

_____

Level 2: Topical steroids

_____

_____

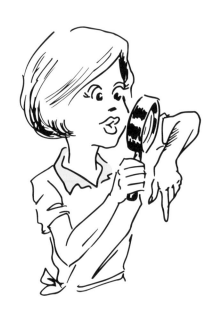

LIVE WITHOUT ECZEMA

The Handbook for Younger Children and their Parents*

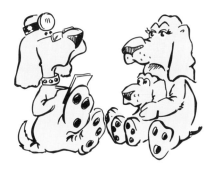

Part 1: Introduction

This approach to the treatment of atopic skin disease is **complementary** rather than **alternative** to conventional treatment. Existing treatment principles are added to, creating a programme that is very effective.

An important aspect of the programme is **behaviour modification** to eliminate the damage caused to skin by scratching. Also emphasized is the relevance of **attitude** and **circumstance**.

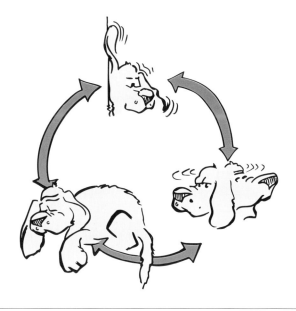

---

*Not for photocopying. Further copies of this handbook can be obtained from the Publisher.

Chronic eczema causes **months and years of misery**. Let's replace all that with only the **days of inconvenience** needed for the effective treatment of acute relapses.

Atopy

Having 'atopy' means being born prone to develop eczema, hay fever and asthma. Hay fever and asthma are allergic conditions, like the rhinitis that is caused in summer by a high pollen count. Eczema is much more to do with dry skin.

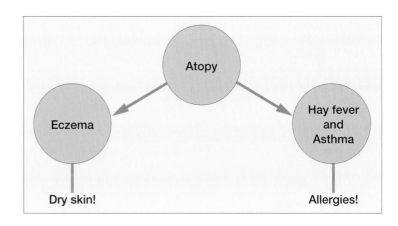

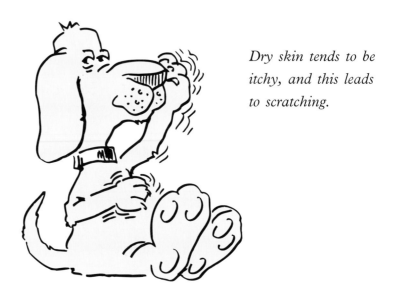

Dry skin tends to be itchy, and this leads to scratching.

Scratching

Even normal skin when scratched will eventually look like chronic eczema under a microscope.

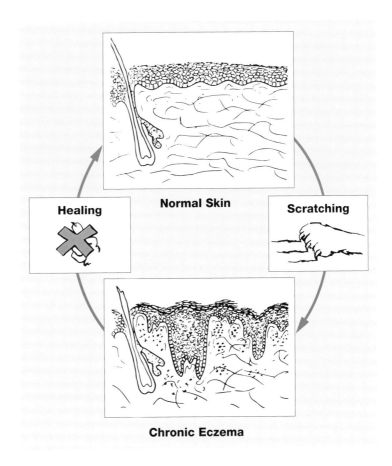

Healing   **Normal Skin**   **Scratching**

Chronic Eczema

> *Healing can only occur if scratching stops*

The Vicious Circle

SO ...

With dryness, itching and scratching a vicious circle is established.

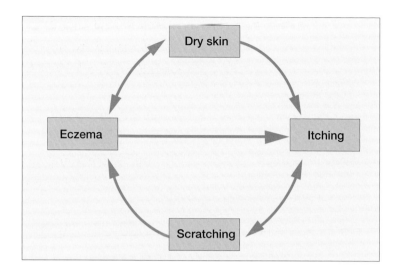

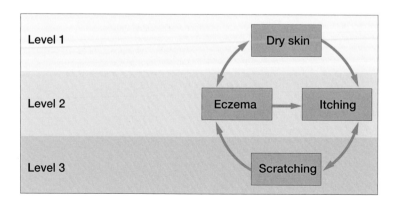

Areas that are easiest
to scratch and rub are
especially susceptible to
chronic eczema.

Breaking the Vicious Circle

The vicious circle of chronic eczema has three levels

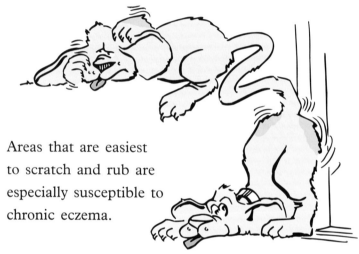

Conventional treatment provides emollients for Level 1 and topical steroids for Level 2 ... BUT **neither are sufficient for Level 3!**

Level 3 needs its own special treatment.

Chronic eczema only heals with all three levels of treatment, as described in The Programme ...

First ... Some general points

Food

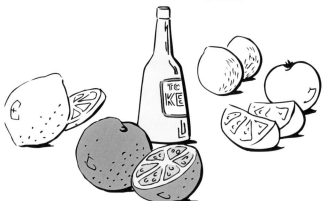

For most children with eczema, what is eaten is not important. It is true that active eczema can worsen with certain foods but this is not allergy — it is a non-specific toxicity. Once the skin has healed the food can be eaten again without any problem.

Thus it has been known from long time that oranges, lemons and tomatoes can give a toxic reaction when eaten. This phenomenon usually disappears with age. Otherwise, it is particularly associated with existing eczema, or recently healed skin — in these phases the skin is relatively unstable.

Infections

Infections such as sore throats can sometimes worsen eczema in a non-specific way.

Clothing

Cotton is always to be preferred to wool and synthetic clothing. The latter can give rise to mechanical irritation and hence itch, on atopic skin.

SITUATIONS, CIRCUMSTANCES AND ACTIVITIES ASSOCIATED WITH SCRATCHING AND RUBBING

Name: _____

Date: _____

1.

2.

3.

4.

5.

6.

Part 2: The Programme

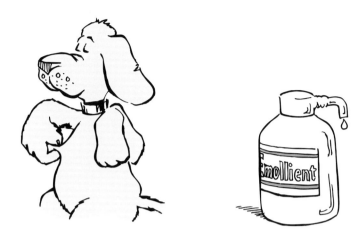

The Vicious Circle and The Three Levels of Treatment

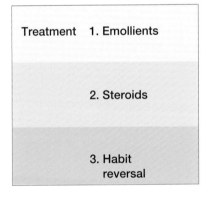

Treatment	1. Emollients
	2. Steroids
	3. Habit reversal

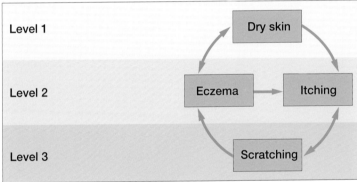

Level 1: Emollients

Atopic skin becomes dry because it is abnormally porous.

Dry skin must be treated with emollient, which prevents water loss and lubricates the skin. It is especially important to use emollients frequently at the beginning of treatment. The more inflamed, thickened and dry the skin is the more often an emollient must be used.

141

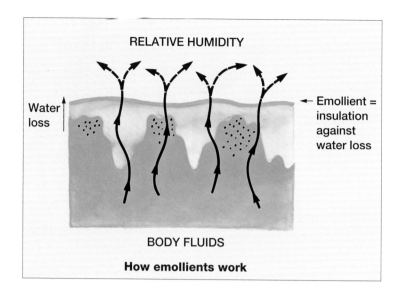

RELATIVE HUMIDITY

Water loss

Emollient = insulation against water loss

BODY FLUIDS

How emollients work

Use Emollients ...

- *Thinly*
- *Gently*
- *Quickly*
- *Frequently*

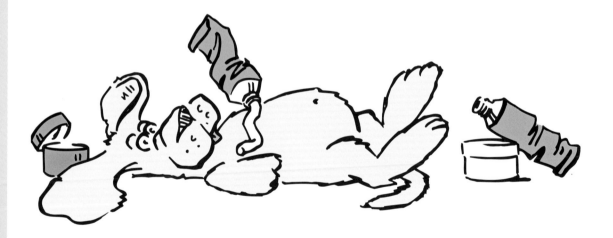

The drying of the skin will be affected by changes in the environment, and bodily function — know when more emollients will be needed!

Level 2: Steroids

Eczema and itch are effectively treated by steroid creams and ointments. The stronger the steroid the more effective it is. Fear of side effects often results in inadequate treatment, with frequent and rapid relapses. Side effects are not seen until after MANY weeks of treatment with strong steroids. There is more risk of developing **chronic** eczema with weak steroids, or with too short a treatment period, than of developing side effects from strong steroids.

How topical steroids work

The healing with topical steroids is in two stages. When the skin first looks good there is still some hidden healing to accomplish:

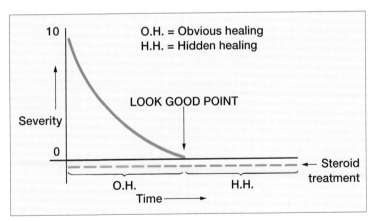

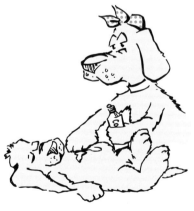

> *Use Steroids ...*
>
> - *As prescribed !*
> - *Don't stop too soon !*

The use of creams

- All topical treatments must be used consistently — in a **planned** way. The application must be brisk and without any unnecessary massage. The steroid should be applied morning and/or evening, and the emollients are used as often as is necessary to prevent the skin from drying.

- The amount of cream that is used depends upon the area treated and how dry the skin is. After treatment the skin should not feel sticky ... **only a shine is required !**

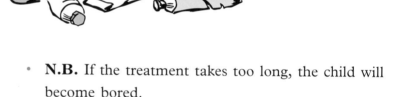

- **N.B.** If the treatment takes too long, the child will become bored.

- Apply the steroid on all areas affected by eczema.

- Then emollient can be put over the whole body, and should be put on again as soon as the skin **begins** to dry. At the beginning of a treatment this could mean one hour after the steroid has been used — later on only once or twice a day.

- Emollients are thus used on areas treated and not treated with steroids. No steroid without emollients, but emollient can be used without steroid.

Level 3: Habits and scratching

When a behaviour is repeated enough it becomes a habit. Although it may originally have been provoked by a particular stimulus, later it becomes linked to other stimuli and circumstances: it generalises. Scratching may begin in new eczema as a response to itch — in long-standing eczema this is often only part of the picture.

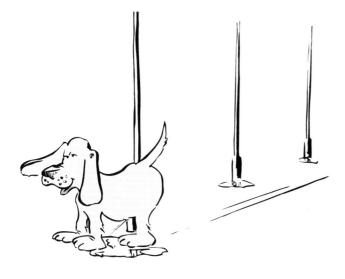

At the same time as generalising, a habit tends to become unconscious.

Thus, children not only scratch because of itch, but because of circumstances. Such situations include when undressing, after a shower or a bath, after topical treatment, watching television and going to bed. Scratching is more noticeable when it starts — when it becomes a habit, both child and parents become **relatively** unaware of the behaviour.

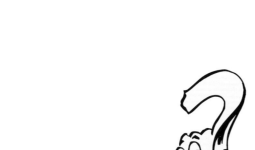

Scratching is sometimes used, consciously or unconsciously, as a form of non-verbal communication — especially within the family.

However, children can easily learn how to change their behaviour ...

Changing behaviour

If we tend to become unaware of bad habits, before we can change them ...

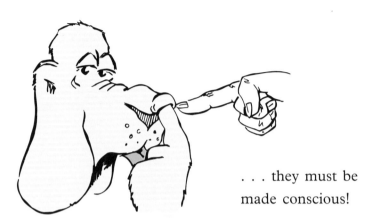

. . . they must be made conscious!

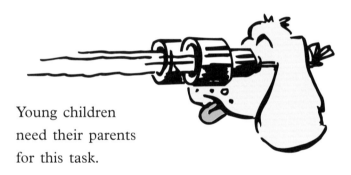

Young children
need their parents
for this task.

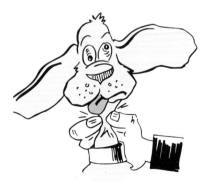

First of all ... Scratching because of itching

Itch can easily be controlled without damaging the skin by teaching the child to PINCH where it is itching, or to press a nail into the skin.

The child will then also have an opportunity to help him/herself.

146

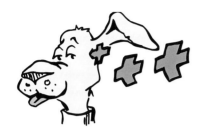

This new behaviour is particularly important at the beginning of treatment as itch is then at its worst.

Reinforce this adaptive response with support and encouragement.

Next ... Scratching because of habit and circumstance

- Introduce new behaviours **incompatible** with scratching and rubbing.

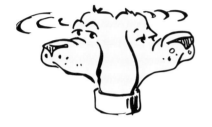

> *Use*
> - *Talk*
> - *Play*
> - *Diversion*
> - *Distraction*

- *Dispense with **unessential** provocative situations for the duration of the programme.*

- *Adapt **essential** difficult activities by*

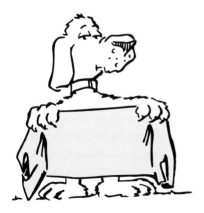

> *Planning ahead*
> *Doing them quickly*
> *Keeping hands busy*

> **So ... Encourage, Innovate, and Anticipate ...**

The programme

Phase One: all three levels

- For the first four days all three levels must be used intensively. Constant supervision is needed day and night.
- A plan is useful. Everyone involved should understand what is required.
- A list of suggestions for Level 3 will be helpful.

Phase two: Levels 1 and 2 especially

- Emollient and topical steroid treatment continues for up to six weeks.
- Gradually vigilance at Level 3 can be relaxed.

Phase 3: Level 1 ... + Vigilance

- Once healing is thorough, only emollient treatment is continued, though not necessarily indefinitely.
- Vigilance for the symptoms and signs of any relapse continues ...

Important rules

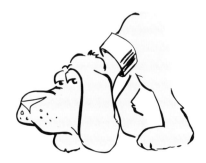

1. Never tell the child to stop scratching.

NEVER say: Stop scratching !!!

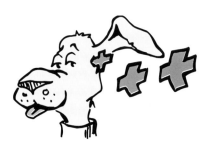

2. Support and encourage adaptive responses.

Give support!

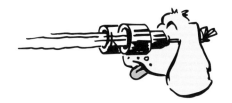

3. Prepare yourself for difficult situations — plan ahead. For example decide what to do after the shower, and topical treatments. Play, talk ...

Be aware of difficult situations

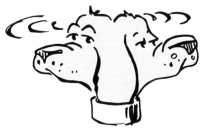

4. Try actively to distract the child if it begins to scratch. Talk, play ...

5. Never put on a cream or ointment later than 20 minutes before going to bed.

6. During the first four days, never leave the child alone, even for a second in difficult situations.

Use distraction

Practical tips

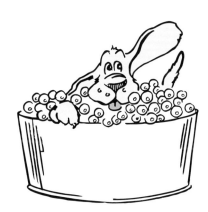

1. Undressing and putting on creams and ointments

The child must not do this alone. Talk and play when undressing the child. Treat quickly. Put on clothes straight away and play with the child intensively for the following 10 minutes.

2. Shower or bath

Undress quickly, take the bath under supervision, pat the skin dry with a towel, put on treatment quickly, do something together.

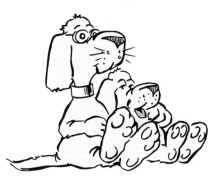

3. Television

Sit with the child, holding its hands.

4. Nights

Night-time scratching diminishes as scratching stops during the day.

TREATMENT SCHEDULE

Name: _____ Date _____

Level 1: Emollients _____
_____
_____

Level 2: Topical steroids _____
_____
_____

Date						
a.m.						
p.m.						

Date						
a.m.						
p.m.						

Level 3 : Habit reversal

Difficult times	*Ways of coping*
1. _____	1. _____
2. _____	2. _____
3. _____	3. _____
4. _____	4. _____
5. _____	5. _____
6. _____	6. _____

Part 3: Follow-up

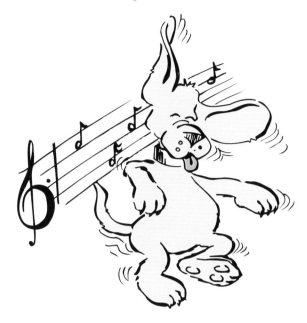

Once healing has been thoroughly accomplished, continue with Level 1 treatment only, as necessary — but beware of relapses!

LOOK at, and **FEEL** the skin daily during convalescence. Recently healed chronic eczema remains unstable for several weeks ...

Think of ...

• *Itchiness*
• *Dryness*
• *Redness*
• *Roughness*

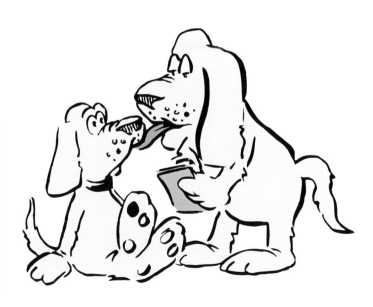

When an acute relapse is identified — **TREAT IT !**

Help STAMP OUT chronic eczema ...

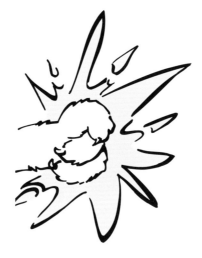

ZAP THE RELAPSE !

Remember!

Itch will go if relapse is treated promptly...

Regime for acute relapse

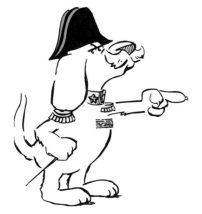

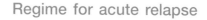

> *3 days steroid twice daily**
> *3 days steroid once daily*
> *plus*
> *Intensive use of emollients*
>
> * Topical steroids which are used once daily can subsequently be
> used on alternate days.

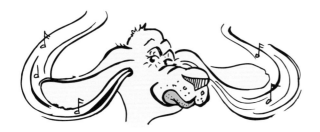

> *No child need*
> *'Live with eczema' ...*
>
> *The aim of treatment is to*
> *'LIVE WITHOUT ECZEMA' !*

As convalescence progresses the skin becomes more stable ...

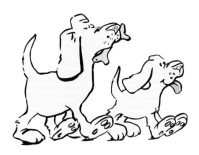

> *Stop using emollients routinely!*
> *Begin to assess the skin routinely!*

Look at the skin

Is there redness, is it dry, rough or itchy?

- The more cautious you are
- The sooner you begin your treatment
- The stronger steroid you use
- The more consistent you are with emollients at the beginning of treatment

Then ...

- The sooner the skin will heal
- The less steroid will be used
- The less trouble you will get with eczema, and with side effects from both eczema and steroids

> **Remember !**
> *Consistent* use of emollients!
> ***Aggressive* use of steroids!**
> *Disciplined* behaviour!

Then there is only the predisposition to eczema to live with.

FOLLOW-UP SCHEDULE

Name: _____

Date: _____

(A) Every day check for

    Redness
    Dryness
    Itchiness
    Roughness

(B) For any relapse treat with

Level 1: Emollients

_____

_____

_____

Level 2: Topical steroids

_____

_____

_____

EMOLLIENTS IN COMMON USE

Creams (in increasing thickness)

Cetomacrogol A
Diprobase
E45
Hydromol
Zinc and castor oil cream 1 part, oily cream 9 parts
Oily cream
Unguentum Merck

Ointments (in increasing thickness)

Liquid paraffin 50% + white soft paraffin 50%
White soft paraffin
Yellow soft paraffin

> *Trial packs containing small amounts of a range of emollients are useful in assessing patient preference.*

Bath additives

Hydromol emollient
Oilatum emollient
Emulsiderm liquid emulsion
Diprobath
Balneum bath oil
Balneum Plus bath oil (contains lauromacrogols)
Oilatum shower gel
Aveeno sachets (oily or regular)

Soap substitutes

Aqueous cream
Emulsifying ointment
Unguentum Merck

For the scalp

Arachis oil
Coconut oil

For the external auditory meatus

Cetamacrogol **carefully** applied with a cotton bud

TOPICAL CORTICOSTEROIDS IN COMMON USE

Grade IV: Mild

Hydrocortisone 0.5% cream/ointment
Hydrocortisone 1% cream/ointment
Hydrocortisone 2.5% cream/ointment

Grade III: Moderate

Eumovate cream/ointment (clobetastone butyrate 0.05%)
Alphaderm cream (Hydrocortisone 1%, urea 10%)

Grade II: Potent

Betnovate cream/ointment/**scalp application** (betamethasone (as valerate) 0.1%)
Cutivate cream (flutisone propionate 0.05%)
Cutivate ointment (flutisone propionate 0.005%)
Diprosone cream/ointment (betamethasone 0.05% (as dipropionate)
Elocon cream/ointment (mometasone furoate 0.1%)
Locoid cream (hydrocortisone butyrate 0.1%)
Metosyn cream/ointment/**scalp lotion** (fluocinonide 0.05%)
Nerisone oily cream (diflucortolone valerate 0.1%)
Propaderm cream/ointment (beclomethasone dipropionate 0.025%)
Synalar cream/ointment/**scalp gel** (fluocinolone acetonide 0.025%)

Grade I: Very Potent

Dermovate cream/ointment/scalp application (clobetasol propionate 0.05%)
Nerisone forte oily cream (diflucortolone valerate 0.3%)

For the external auditory meatus

Betamethasone sodium phosphate 0.1% drops

THREE GOLDEN RULES FOR DEALING WITH STRESS

1 Regular Relaxation

- Choose a favourite technique and practise it frequently: e.g. yoga, meditation, relaxation exercises, t'ai chi, self-hypnosis or music.

- If it suits you, use exercise to relax: e.g. cycling, skating, dancing, power-walking, swimming or aerobics.

2 Balance Life

- Review your life-style and ensure each domain has enough emphasis: home and family, work and colleagues, leisure and friends.

- Distinguish between what can and cannot be done. Agree rather than disagree. Stop before you are tired. Ask someone to help.

3 Avoid Bad Habits

- Beware and respect the effects of caffeine, tobacco, alcohol, tranquillisers and sleeping pills.

- Ensure you have a sensible and healthy diet. Enjoy regular and adequate sleep.

PRIMARY CARE INFORMATION SHEET

The Combined Approach ('Habit Reversal') for Atopic Skin Disease

- The approach was introduced in 1989 at the Daniel Turner Clinic, Westminster Hospital. For out-patients with atopic eczema, it combines conventional topical treatment with a behaviour modification technique called **habit reversal**. This procedure aims to eliminate self-damaging behaviours characteristic of chronic eczema, such as repetitive scratching and rubbing. The Combined Approach is suitable both for children and adults.

- All referrals from general practitioners are first assessed dermatologically before being considered appropriate for the Combined Approach. The programme then requires a series of appointments for: Assessment, Introduction of treatment, Review of treatment, and Follow-up.

  From assessment to beginning follow-up takes between five and seven weeks. Follow-up can continue for several months with appointments at six weeks, three and six months.

- The Combined Approach aims to educate all patients in the rationale for and the appropriate use of emollients and topical steroids. In addition, following a week's measurement of the frequency of self-damaging behaviour, **habit reversal** procedures are taught. Throughout the programme there is an emphasis on positive self-care, and the avoidance of risk factors.

- The Combined Approach eliminates the chronic syndrome of long-standing atopic skin disease. Patients then only require intermittent treatment of acute relapses, using a treatment schedule that can easily be followed in primary health care. Both patient and general practitioner receive written advice on the required procedures. Further advice is available at follow-up.

USEFUL UK ADDRESSES

For self-help literature

National Eczema Society
163 Eversholt Street
London
NW1 1BU

Tel: 0171 388 4097

For hand tally-counters

FKI Cableform Ltd
ENM
Gratix Works
Gratix Lane
Sowerby Bridge
West Yorkshire
HX6 2PH

Tel: 01422 833 533

For house dust mite proof bed linen

Allerbreathe
S. Devon & Cornwall Institute for the Blind
Stonehouse
Plymouth
Devon
PL1 3PE

Tel: 01752 662 317

REFERENCES AND FURTHER READING

Atopic Skin Disease

Hanifin, J.M. and Rajka, G. (1980). Diagnostic features of atopic dermatitis. *Acta Dermatol-Venereologica* **92** (Suppl.), 44–47.

Rajka, G. (1989). *Essential Aspects of Atopic Dermatitis.* Springer Verlag, Berlin.

Ruzicka, T., Ring, S. and Przybilla, B. (Eds) (1991). *Handbook of Atopic Eczema.* Springer Verlag, Berlin.

Williams, H.C. (1995). On the definition and epidemiology of atopic dermatitis. *Dermatology Clinics* **13**, 649–657.

Management in General

Bridgett, C. (1995). *Live Without Eczema* (video). Medical Illustration Group, Charing Cross and Westminster Hospital, London.

Loden, M. (1995). Biophysical properties of dry atopic and normal skin with special reference to the effects of skin care products. *Acta Dermatol-Venereologica* **192** (Suppl.), 1–48.

McHenry, P.M. Williams, H.C. and Bingham E.A. (1995). Management of atopic eczema. *British Medical Journal* **310**, 843–847.

Surber, C. Itin, P.H. Bircher, A.J. and Maibach, H.I. (1995). Topical corticosteroids. *Journal of the American Academy Dermatology* **32**, 1025–1030.

Habit Reversal

Azrin, N.H. and Nunn, R.G. (1973). Habit reversal: a method of eliminating nervous habits and tics. *Behaviour Research & Therapy* **II**, 619–628.

Ehlers, A. Stangier, U. and Gieler, U (1995). Treatment of atopic dermatitis: a comparison of psychological and dermatological approaches to relapse prevention. *Journal of Consulting and Clinical Psychology* **63**, 624–634.

Goldblum, R.W. and Piper, W.N. (1954). Artificial lichenification produced by a scratching machine. *Journal of Investigative Dermatology* **22**, 405–445.

Melin, L., Frederiksen, T., Norén, P. and Swebilius, B.G. (1986). Behavioural treatment of scratching in patients with atopic dermatitis. *British Journal of Dermatology* **115**, 467–474.

Naylor, P.F.D. (1955). The reaction to friction of patients with flexural eczema. *British Journal of Dermatology* **67**, 385–391.

Norén, P. (1995). Habit reversal: a turning point in the treatment of atopic dermatitis. *Clinical and Experimental Dermatology* **20**, 2–5.

Norén, P. and Melin, L. (1989). The effect of combined topical steroids and habit–reversal treatment in patients with atopic dermatitis. *British Journal of Dermatology* **121**, 359–366

Rubin, L. (1949). Hyperkeratosis in response to mechanical irritation. *Journal of Investigative Dermatology* **13**, 313–315.

INDEX

163